ROSIE

ROSIE:
THE INVESTIGATION OF
A WRONGFUL DEATH

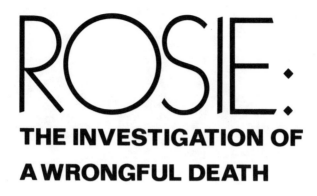

by Ellen Frankfort

with Frances Kissling

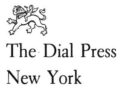

The Dial Press

New York

Published by
The Dial Press
1 Dag Hammarskjold Plaza
New York, New York 10017

Manufactured in the United States of America

First printing

Design by Karin Batten

Library of Congress Cataloging in Publication Data

Frankfort, Ellen.
    Rosie: the investigation of a wrongful death.

    1. Abortion services—United States—Finance.
2. Medicaid—United States. 3. Death—Causes.
4. Jimenez, Rosaura. 5. Abortion—Texas.
I. Kissling, Frances, 1943–   joint author.
II. Title.
HQ767.5.U5F72   362.1'9'880926   79–861
ISBN 0–8037–7504–0

This book is dedicated to the memory of Rosie
and the women of McAllen

CONTENTS

A wrongful death: The statute usually provides that an action can be instituted by the beneficiary of the decedent for any wrongful act, neglect, or default which causes death.

—Prosser Texts 902
(Fourth edition, 1971)

◆ ◆ ◆

The family of Rosie Jimenez is filing a wrongful-death suit against Maria Pineda; Joseph A. Califano, Jr., HEW; and the Texas State Department of Health.

E.F.

ROSIE

INTRODUCTION

"Did you or didn't you?" the doctor asked.

Rosie tried to respond, but it hurt too much. She lifted her arm toward her throat.

"Do you want to tell us something?" the doctor asked, noting her effort to get at the tubing coming out of her neck. "You are very sick; you may not pull through. It would make it easier to treat you if you told us the truth." And then lowering his voice, the doctor said, "We're not here to punish you. We want to do all we can to help you."

Pauline wasn't sure if Rosie could feel anything, but she kept on massaging her legs. It was hard to look at her. She was a dark greenish-brown and there was blood coming from her eyes. Pauline was surprised Rosie was still conscious. She had been in this state for six days and had survived two operations. The doctors would not say anything definite.

But that smell. Pauline remembered it. It was the same smell her father gave off as he lay dying.

Again Rosie made a move toward her throat.

The doctor sat down on the bed next to her. "You don't have to talk," he said, as he placed her hand between his own. "Just squeeze once if you did and twice if you didn't." He waited. Pauline looked away. Very slowly he repeated, "Once if you did, Rosie, and twice if you did not." The doctor was beaming. "Just what I thought," he said. Then looking up, he added, "That's a good girl, Rosie. Thank you."

Pauline turned to Rosie again. She detected the same feeble

movement toward her neck. "Rosie, Rosie, do you have something more to say?" she asked. She thought she saw Rosie nod.
She also thought tears were coming from her eyes. But it was hard
to tell. Pauline took a pad she saw lying on the night table and
tore off a sheet. The word *penicillin* was printed on top. "Here,
Rosie, write down what you want to say."

Rosie took the piece of paper and a pen. Pauline helped prop
her up so she could write. It took a while to steady herself, but
she was able to scribble some words before the pen fell from her
hand. Pauline helped her back into position and straightened out
the sheet. The paper was lying on her chest. Pauline lifted it to
the light above the bed. She could not understand the writing.
The first word looked like *Please.* There was a *me* and another
word that started with a *p.* "Please . . . me . . . p . . ." Pauline
looked carefully at the last word. She got it. *P e a c e.* Now the
sentence fell into place. "Please let me die in peace." Pauline
turned her head so Rosie would not see the tears.

As a student of philosophy, I was taught to be cautious when
it came to causal connections. One event may follow another, but
is not necessarily caused by it. Chance, coincidence, a third and
prior unknown circumstance can as easily link two events as
causality. Skeptical by temperament, I had scant difficulty in
accepting these lessons. Therefore when Frances Kissling, who
was then the executive director of the National Abortion Federation, informed me on October 28, 1977, that the first woman had
died because of the cutback of Medicaid funds for abortion, I
reacted with prudence.

Politically, it was tempting to react otherwise: the dead woman
—poor, the mother of a four-year-old girl—was in addition Hispanic. With these "credentials," she seemed irresistibly correct as
a feminist martyr.

When Frances told me of the October 3 death, we were on our
way to a party celebrating another first—a novel written by an
unknown middle-aged woman.

With the notion that all progress, indeed, all historical precedents are accompanied by some sacrifice, I quietly passed along the news of the Mexican-American mother. "Medicaid-related" was how I worded the connection between the cutoff of government funding and the death.

The response was immediate—"Let's take some action." One writer, Alix Kates Shulman, asked me if I knew about the meetings women were holding to plan a November 12 demonstration at New York University Law School to protest an award being given to Secretary of Health, Education and Welfare, Joseph Califano.

On the appointed evening, I joined a group of women at the law school. Some were professors, some students; several had small babies whom they diapered on a large conference table, laying out the safety pins and Pampers with an ease once reserved for legal-size memo pads. Most had not heard of the death in Texas, and my brief report was received with ambivalent awe. Now the demonstration had taken on more significance, but it came at the cost of a woman's life.

Quickly, the women shifted from the hypothetical to the actual. Califano could no longer be asked what would happen *if* a woman died after Medicaid funds were cut off. A woman had died. We wanted to know how he felt to be partially responsible. It would not do to echo Jimmy Carter: "Life is not fair."

In light of the government's policy, Califano might state that death is unfair and law professors uninformed. Every citizen does *not* have the right to life, liberty, and happiness. The right to life is for those with money, not those with Medicaid cards. Of course, not one of us thought Califano capable of such a fierce honesty and counted, instead, on jolting him into an awareness of the callousness of his policy by a solemn moment of mourning.

We don't know if he was jolted. He never came out to face the two thousand women and men who surrounded the law school and spilled over into Washington Square Park.

But the rest of the nation saw them. The television-network crews, perched atop large vans, cameras and lights ready, zoomed in on the large gathering of women who were chanting "murderer." That night, millions of Americans watched as Califano hid inside the law school, unwilling to answer the charge of murder.

The New York demonstration a success, feminists planned similar ones throughout the country, hoping that Califano, like Lyndon Johnson at the height of the Vietnam War protests, would find himself sufficiently reviled to consider resigning. And as if that were not enough, *The New York Times* ran an editorial, less explicit in its charges, but suggesting a similar link between the cutoff of Medicaid funds for abortion and the subsequent death.

With a simplicity in keeping with mourning, the editorial was captioned "First Victim." It began,

> Last month, a 27-year-old Mexican-American, the unwed mother of a 4-year-old child, died in a hospital in McAllen, Texas, from complications caused by a cheap abortion in a nearby Mexican border town. The dead woman carried a Medicaid card, but it did her little good. On Aug. 4, the Federal government had stopped paying for abortions for the poor unless the life of the mother is endangered. The woman's life presumably was not in danger—not until she went across the border and paid $40 to terminate an unwanted pregnancy. Legal abortions performed in McAllen, Texas, are a lot more expensive than that.

With a decorum in keeping with the *Times,* the editorial ended with a suggested course of reflection: "Congress should use the time to ponder the consequences of the present policy. The Government cannot stop abortions. It can only stop paying for them."

How had the death of an unknown woman become a public issue?

Two weeks after she died, Dr. Daniel Chester, who had treated her in the hospital, phoned the Center for Disease Control in Atlanta. He informed them of a cluster of five abortion complications, including two highly unusual cases in the tetanus family. One of them happened to be the fatal case.

Within the CDC, a division of HEW, is the Abortion Surveillance Branch of the Family Planning Evaluation Division, Bureau of Epidemiology.

After consulting with the Texas Department of Health, the Abortion Surveillance Branch, at the request of the State of Texas, sent two doctors, one of them female—"junior officers" in the CDC's military parlance—to McAllen, where they interviewed Dr. Chester, a Planned Parenthood official, and the dead woman's personal physician. The two CDC doctors, members of the Epidemiological Investigation Service, were then joined by a CDC colleague who was on assignment to the Texas Department of Health in Austin. Together the team reviewed the hospital records and talked with health officials from Mexico City and Tamaulipas State (which includes the "nearby Mexican border town," Reynosa), a Reynosa doctor, an El Paso health official, and the dead woman's cousin, a hospital orderly. Except for the Planned Parenthood official, all the interviewees were male; and except for the Planned Parenthood official and the cousin, all were doctors.

The team's findings were published in the CDC's *MMWR, The Morbidity and Mortality Weekly Report* (Mortality in this sense means death. Morbidity means major complications.): "This is the first confirmed illegal abortion-related death reported to the CDC since February 2, 1976," said an editorial note, adding: "Not all states have discontinued public financing of abortions, but . . . Texas withdrew financial support for abortions after federal support was withdrawn on August 4."

There was a quick backlash based on a single article in a medical trade magazine *Ob. Gyn. News.* "Doubts Arise about Abortion Martyr" ran a headline in the *Washington Post.* On November 28, staff writer Bill Peterson wrote: "A woman portrayed as a martyr when she died from an illegal abortion after Medicaid funds were cut off may simply have been trying to keep her pregnancy secret when she slipped across the border to have the operation performed in the back of a Mexican pharmacy."

On the same day the *Post* ran its story, the *Boston Globe* ran a piece by Robert Toth of the *Los Angeles Times:* "Serious doubt has been raised about a widely reported allegation that a Mexican-American woman, who died after crossing the Texas border in September for a Mexican abortion, went there because of a cutoff in Federal Medicaid funds."

Charges and countercharges became more frequent, and the controversy appeared to be escalating. Although I planned and participated in demonstrations, and even spoke on TV about "the poor Chicana," that skepticism, early and deeply ingrained, would not go away.

I decided to look into the matter myself. Armed with the skeleton of facts, fleshed out in a conflicting body of interpretation, I took off for Texas. I wanted to get a sense of the woman's life, and I felt there was no way to know whether the Medicaid cutback had actually led to her death unless I talked to someone who knew her.

I stopped in Atlanta to speak with CDC officials; I had hoped to learn from them the name of the dead woman. But in keeping with CDC policy, they kept it a secret. I came away with little more than the skimpy facts first reported.

Not once did it occur to me that the facts themselves, coming straight from official documents, could be wrong.

PART 1

FEELING MY WAY, KNOWING NOTHING

ONE THE SETTING

McAllen is a small town on the southernmost tip of Texas. Like most small towns, it has a way of suggesting thwarted aspiration. Rexall may boast the best hamburger in town; you may still be able to find a full-length ladies' slip with a trim of heart-shaped antique ivory lace topping a rayon garment in a light coral color that approximates unblemished flesh; and at least one shoe salesman is living out his life making sure both feet get measured before a single shoe is shown, reminding you, as he kneels to adjust the lever which locks each foot into its proper size, that the left is always a trifle longer than the right. Human nature, he remarks, as he picks up a hook-shaped pole to secure the box that contains the pair best fitted to your feet.

Outside the store are parking spots set at neat diagonals to the curb. They are rarely full. The absence of traffic and the blinking yellow lights make Main Street a pleasant thoroughfare to drive along if you want to get from one end of town to the other without ever coming to a full stop.

No matter Main Street is fading. For all its archetypal turn-of-the-century, small-town markers, McAllen is no ordinary American town. It sits quietly, even deceptively, a mere seven miles from Mexico.

Stepping off Texas International Flight 916, passengers from Houston are greeted by a sign, HUNTERS CLAIM GUNS AT BAGGAGE COUNTER. Three small palm trees at the entrance to the arrival lounge sway in the mild gusts whipped up by the landings and take-offs. Inside are courtesy phones for the local hotels: Ramada

Inn, Rodeway Inn, Royal Palm Motel, Happy Landing Motel, Hilton Inn, Palmview Golf Motel, and La Posada, which advertises itself as "a special place in time. Ten minutes from Reynosa's International Bridge into Mexico, La Posada offers you a unique blend of twentieth-century American convenience with eighteenth-century charm. For your comfort, two hundred twenty-five beautiful guest rooms, seven suites, two restaurants, gift and package store, free parking, heated swimming pool, landscaped, cloistered patio, and the exciting Tesoro Club. Complete banquet and meeting facilities also available. Bienvenidos."

Who comes to McAllen, I wonder, as I walk over to National and Budget Car Rentals and call out, "Which one of you is cheaper?" Two men in cowboy hats let out a hearty chuckle. National has no one waiting. I get its rate, then do a quick check with Budget. There is no difference. Soon the glass exit door, with a small blue plaque showing two trees and the words, WELCOME, MCALLEN, CITY OF PALMS, opens automatically. In my hands are the keys to the car and a map showing how to get from the airport to La Posada Hotel.

I take note of the Rose Lawn Perpetual Care Burial Park coming up on my right. It is a sedate-looking place, nothing ostentatious, nothing neglected. The granite gravestones bear solid Yankee names: Duncan, Williams, Phillips. It seems unlikely she is here being perpetually cared for.

Main Street ends at a railroad crossing. But there is no need to stop, look, and listen. Trains no longer run through McAllen. As if to mock the defunct tracks, trucks labeled "land trains" jut out from the lonesome row of warehouses linked to one another like nameless roadside diners.

The rigs, their rear ends maneuvered into the large barnlike openings, rest severed from their cabs. Inside the warehouses, carrots, a competitive orange to the shiny painted shafts and troughs, are separated from their grassy greens, the men hosing down the earth's daily yield while the women stand waiting to place the cleansed carrots into clear plastic bags.

Susie's Carrots. You can't miss them up in New York's Grand Union; they're in the only bag of produce with a photo—a picture of Susie when she was six. Susie, the twenty-seven-year-old daughter of the warehouse owner. For four days the carrots will endure the trip north, the smile of Susie to keep them from rotting.

TEXAS LAW REQUIRES ALL BEER SALES TO BE STRICTLY ON A CASH BASIS reads the sign posted on the door of the warehouse next to Susie's Carrots. The trucks in front, ready to go, are painted a golden beer brown with JAX in red letters on each truck.

Across the railroad tracks from JAX is a one-story stucco, pastel-pink entertainment hall. The sign outside says nothing concerning the manner of payment, only that there is no cover charge. A cocktail costs one dollar; a beer, fifty cents. That is, if you get there on weekdays and come before ten. To the right of the Pink Panther is a silver sports car. The sun bounces off its back, making it look like a low-lying metal mushroom, all aglow.

At any point along the stretch of warehouses lining Business Highway 83, two terra-cotta cupolas can be seen transcending the landscape, architectural appendices—lookouts from which to behold groves of oranges, grapefruits, flat fertile fields, built in an era when only a train whistle could puncture the quiet of a cloistered patio where trays of *huevos rancheros* appeared after dawn, set out by servants as silent as the Sisters of Charity; before Susie's Carrots came along and offered up noise, plastic bags, late-night shifts, and one dollar an hour; before the Great Western Chain bought up the old Spanish mansion, removed the southern moss, exposed a white stucco made stark by paint, polished the tiles, placed a pool in the patio, and lit up the joint, newly named La Posada, with enough floods and spots to thrill a first-night audience.

I check into La Posada with haste. I am anxious to have a swim at the end of this day which I liken to the Sabbath—a day for absorption and reflection before the real work begins. All I must do is hand over my American Express—the card that has carried me to this spot—and sign in.

When I was a teen-ager, there was a plastic surgeon who redid noses. Girls with long noses, bent noses, knobby noses, would return after a holiday with all excess cartilage gone, sheared off by a scalpel. In its stead stood a pinched little button tilted upward. The Kopp Nose, it came to be called. With time, a nose might drop or the tip turn purple long after the initial puffiness subsided. Without extra charge, the doctor would cut again until he carved out a perfect Kopp Nose, recognizable to all, regardless of the face, by the tiny lines he left that traced the path of his knife; it was a signature of sorts, proof the job had been done, the nose renovated.

The interior of La Posada brings into mind the Kopp Nose: a wrought-iron stairwell, its curving steps covered with red carpet, spirals up to the Tesoro Club right in the middle of the lobby. The Spanish-style chairs have maroon velvet cushions, a bit too new; and the dark wooden frames look too regal to be real. They are favored by the elderly retirees who look as though they are waiting for a noonday whistle to announce a lunchtime break. It is quiet, except for the muffled conversation of two young men with shades and lots of cowboy leather.

My room is fine. Double beds with red and black heavy cotton print spreads with black fringe on the bottom, a suitcase rack supported by leather straps, and full-length French doors opening onto a patio. On either side of the doors is a high-backed chair with a seat woven of straw, placed so as to leave undisturbed the symmetry of the arcade that wraps around the inner courtyard. The angle of the arch, along with the chairs, serves as an invisible divider, defining each guest's area while adding an illusion of private domain.

Beyond the arcade, in the center of the patio and to the right of the pool, is a multitiered fountain. The sprays from the smallest jets reach out to the pool below, which in turn overflows onto the one below it. Liquid spokes of invisible umbrellas converge in a stagnant body of still water.

Nothing hard, nothing sharp; circles softened, ceilings made to undulate with archways; architecture from an era when to scallop a circle was to diminish the heat of the sun.

The "winter Texans" have moved from the lobby and are now stretched out on the black and white vinyl bars of the poolside chaises, staring into the steam rising from the heated aqua water. I have seen people in their late sixties and seventies sitting on Broadway benches, waiting for a touch of sun as pigeons strut between the feet that rest on the subway grates below. I have seen them huddled against apartment walls in Brighton Beach, Miami Beach, and Far Rockaway. How different these older people who winter in McAllen! They do not talk. Here, in this Miami for Midwesterners, when they retire to the earth, they take their secrets along with them. With a stubborn dignity and a recalcitrant pride, these older men and women sit alone, their visors over their eyes, their palms together, their backs upright, waiting for a person to make a splash in the water, waiting for something of significant deviation to encourage commentary.

Pam Dee is lifting her face toward the ceiling of the Tesoro Club. Her feet stomp away at the abbreviated electric organ; her eyes are closed, and she is smiling as if in the spell of a supernatural power. The last rays of sun are coming through the large arched window of the cocktail lounge, lighting up one corner of the pool outside.

The cocktail waitress, a tall dark-haired young woman in black stockings and a skirt barely covering her thighs, appears with drinks ordered by the five retirees and myself gathered before dinner. The aqua pool below glistens like holy water.

"*Who* comes to McAllen?" she repeats as she sets a *margarita* in front of me. "Man, no one who has any choice. I'll tell you that much."

"What brought you here?" I ask.

"I was in Colorado, and then my old man got a job down here. As soon as I left Colorado to join him, he met someone else. I'm just doing my time until I can get out."

We chat about her life. I learn that "the other woman" works at the Rose Monocle. "It's easy to spot her. Just look for the ugliest waitress there," she says and walks right through the light arranged for Pam Dee, an insolent sail cutting a sunset cone.

"I'm going to tell you something," she says when she returns, lifting the empty glass from the fake felt coaster. "This is the same country that killed Janis. I'm getting out of here as soon as I can. This place is death. What are y'all doing down here?"

"I'm working on a story. In fact, it's about a young woman who died right in this town."

"What's her name?"

"I don't know her name."

"How can you do a story on someone if you don't know their name?"

"I'm going to find it out. Check out the obits in the town paper. I know her age and the day she died."

"Well, lots of luck," she says, as she collects the cocktail tray.

The seven-mile stretch from Main Street, McAllen, to Mexico, so bountiful with color, is a cornucopia of fear.

Everywhere are warnings. Small shacks with large signs urge drivers to take out special auto insurance before entering Mexico; border banks urge Americans to deposit their cash before crossing. Manmade markers delineate the two lands here in the valley, home of the citrus, where the visible growth is not grapefruit.

Oh, there's an occasional stand, propped up by dust against the unrelenting flatness of the open fields. And if you care to stop, you can purchase a bag with three dozen Ruby Reds for one dollar, the very same grapefruit that costs ninety-five cents a half, back in the hotel coffee shop.

En route to Reynosa I stop at the Family Shopping Center to pick up film. There is a light drizzle. I pull up beside a Studebaker with a rear window made of plastic. It is conspicuous among the pickup trucks and trailers which come in every size; their common link, a penchant for all-letter license plates, a word to distinguish a home whose sole root is a set of wheels.

Traveling along the seven-mile stretch, I pass a cluster of wooden shacks that lean at various angles to the land. They, too, have plastic for windows but are rooted to the earth by cinder blocks. They are the first homes that look like classic migrant shacks from the pages of Steinbeck. Although tiny, they seem hallucinatory—a poor settlement on the tilt, arising out of nowhere.

Texas has a talent for surreal landscapes. NASA, too, looms out of nowhere, a futuristic city of cylinders and domes facing upward like contemporary cathedrals against the endless flat backdrop.

At the International Bridge to Reynosa, there is traffic congestion; it looks like New Yorkers leaving town before a long summer weekend. Except that the traffic here consists of pickup trucks; a few are shiny red, most are purplish blue. All are rimmed with dust. I decide to park the car (I have ignored all warnings about auto insurance) and cross the border by foot. In defiance of the sign cautioning drivers that parking is for shoppers only, I pull into El Rio Andy's and leave the car.

I once did cross a border—the Mexican border—by car.

I was traveling on the "divorce plane" from New York in 1963. All the women on the flight were met in El Paso and driven across the border to Juarez, where we lazed at a poolside patio of a new motel, swapped tales about our soon to be "exes" and bought liquor for little money. (I obliged my "roommate" and bought her four quarts. She invited me to the "divorce party" she was planning.) I remember signing some documents in a Mexican court the next morning about an hour before the flight departed. The crossing from married to unmarried was as unceremonious as going from El Paso to Juarez.

This time I observe the border—the narrow muddy stream that makes the word *river* seem grandiose. The Ku Klux Klan, I've been told, patrols the banks of the Rio Grande looking for submerged bodies of Mexicans trying to slip through the brown water that separates their country from sewerage systems, education, social security. Trains and passports, once the tools of the alien, have been confiscated; VISA and American Express now belong to the vocabulary of commerce.

According to a local tourist magazine, Reynosa "is now a flourishing metropolis of approximately 200,000 population and is the petroleum center of Northeastern Mexico (Petroleoas, Mexicanos, PEMEX). Other industries include cattle, agriculture, manufacturing and a tourist trade." But not a mention of the industry for which Reynosa is known by the women of the Rio Grande Valley, the industry that has brought me to this crossing.

"Nationality?" the border patrol calls out.

"American."

"Go right through," he says, motioning to the turnstiles.

On a lane bearing traffic in the opposite direction, Mexicans —mainly women with children—are lined up, waiting to get into the immigration office. Those inside sit in rows of plastic chairs looking more resigned than angry. I pay the ten-cent toll leading to the bridge.

> WARNING. Pot Users. On your Return Do Not Bring Marijuana into the United States. The Sentence for Smuggling Marijuana is 5 YEARS CONFINEMENT.

It's the first greeting Americans receive. I have been careful; I do not want to go to jail, even for a day.

Young Mexican boys who appear to be about ten are selling cigarettes. They move back and forth quickly alongside the patient crawl of the pickup trucks. I stare through the hurricane-wire mesh, curled on top with an angry barb, to get a glimpse of the Mexican side. There are a few goats tied to a muddy bank, some youngsters running up and down, and trees protruding at unexpected angles. A shabby pastoral setting painted before perspective was discovered.

"I thought it's supposed to be hot in Mexico," a woman behind me remarks.

"It is *supposed* to be," her companion confirms.

At this point, Mexico and McAllen are approximately a block apart. The temperature in McAllen is forty-five. Probably two retired schoolteachers with the black line of an atlas border still stuck in their heads.

I stop to let them pass. A young Mexican boy dances in front of them, slowly moving backward, motioning them toward him with a maraca in each hand. He gives the maracas a shake and one of the women stops to unsnap the gold latch of her black bag. She offers him some change. "No, dollars," he says. He is not begging; he is performing. He does not want their pennies. He knows that the "winter Texans," the "snowbirds," that his country's shrewder businessmen squawk *"bienvenidos"* to, cross the bridge every day in search of new ways to spend their retirement dollars. Without Reynosa and the border, there would be nothing but El Central Mall, El Rio Andy's, and La Plaza Shopping Center where one can purchase a bag of Ruby Reds right next to a color TV.

Have you ever tried to conceptualize death—what it is like to cease to be forever? Walking from one nation to another, I find nationality as abstract as death. The brown water below does not look treacherous to swim; far less intimidating than the swirling currents of the East River or the filmy pollution of the Hudson. I am trying to absorb the concept of border, what it means to be born on the other side. I watch the young boy reject the pennies handed to him by the ladies, with an aggressive shake of the maracas.

If you are born on one side, you dance on a bridge when you are young, scorned for your hustling and pitied for your need by those born on the other. All your life you have to prove that you deserve to be given something, that you really are industrious, resourceful, ambitious, want to work, go to school, drive a car, raise a family, put money in a bank.

But where do you start if you want to get from the pastoral to the neon? You can scream at the goats that life is unfair or you can strangle aspiration before it takes hold, before you think of jumping in at night and praying, as you hold your breath under water, that you will make it across the river alive.

"Cheap, cheap," the young hustlers call out, holding up cigarette cartons, as soon as I step onto the Mexican side. I shake my head no; they continue to rock back and forth, waiting for another customer. I pass the shops full of Mexican pottery, straw baskets, tin lamps, leather boots, hot-pink ponchos, black lace serapes, stopping only at the liquor store. A quart of Kahlua for $3.50. Tequila Gold for $1.29. Oso Negro, one-hundred-proof vodka, for $1.20. Booze is still a good buy.

On the streets of Reynosa a mother sits, her baby in a shawl attached to her arm like a splint. Her wrinkled hand is held out, but it is too passive for American tastes. The young boys with smooth skin don't invoke guilt. The tourists pass by the motionless hand.

"Did you see how she just sits there in the chill with her baby," comment a couple. The mother gets no sympathy from them. Nor money.

In the Central Plaza a new church has been built next to the old; its entrance, a gaudy imitation of a McDonald's golden arch, is flanked by two tall rectangular columns that do not diminish in diameter as they reach toward the sky. The tiny slits of stained glass look like punch-outs on a computer card.

I come across Calle Diaz, a street dense with medical activity. This is where the dead woman must have gone. According to a Texas Planned Parenthood official, she had her abortion at a drugstore called Guadlupena. The offices along the street look like H & R Block outposts. In one, a skeleton of a hand made of plaster serves as an ashtray. The tops of the two-story stucco buildings are a faded aqua, and out of the windows hang ancient air conditioners. The exhaust fumes from the oversized iron boxes remain trapped in the narrow streets, mingling with those from the cars parked in front of the double meters. Every spot is filled.

Continuing down the narrow crowded street, I pass a window lined with rows of teeth. Next to the dentist is a reducing salon: *"cintura, abdomen, piernas, cadera, espalda,"* can be replaced, rebuilt, reduced. Around the corner is a glass window with the words *Drug Store* written on a golden slant like a gift ribbon. The same ornate lettering spells out *Guadlupena* across the top.

Beyond the display window filled with blond dolls, the inside is dim and looks like the scene of an urgent departure—glass cabinets partly opened, imprints of hands disturbing the smooth layer of dust on which lie syringes, rubber tubing, and vials of pills.

CERRADO is stamped on a white official paper pasted on the door with the date 1-16-78. "Closed." This, I've been told, is where she had the abortion.

"Why is it closed?" I ask a Mexican who appears to be directing traffic in front of the drugstore. *"No comprendo,"* he shrugs.

"Emergencia. Abortar," I say, pointing to my abdomen. He nods and motions for me to follow him as he leaves his post. We walk across the street, past the offices of a dentist, a radiologist, and an emergency surgeon. Their signs jut out like rickety canopies, as oversized as the air conditioners above them.

Between the office of a cardiologist and Universal Radio and Television Store is a narrow alley. It is filled with tanks of gas, old seats from cars, the top part of a shopping cart, a rusty Coke machine without wheels, boxes of empty bottles, a wooden door-frame, shells for fluorescent lights, car tires without treads, and a water-stiffened mop—an inventory of truncated limbs and dissected parts for an anatomy class in American know-how.

A woman comes to the door of a house at the end of the alley. She and the man confer while I wait silently. Seventy-five dollars. With my hand, I gesture no. Forty, she calls out as I start to retreat. No dollars. *Mañana.* Okay? *Comprendo?* She nods and I leave.

Is this where she went instead? Down this alley to abort?

At the corner is a large pharmacy. Inside a young man is mopping up. The Farmacia Paris looks like a small supermarket with its section of hi-fi's, cameras, and TVs. I ask a woman behind the counter why the Guadlupena is closed. She motions to the boy who comes over, mop in hand. I explain that I am in trouble and need an abortion. Not here, the woman says, never. They have all taken note of CERRADO.

Toward the end of Calle Diaz, an office for *emergencias* stands adjacent to a boutique for wedding gowns. I spot another pharmacy, this one seedier looking than the Paris; it has no name. I go inside and explain. The man takes out a syringe and asks for five dollars. But first, he says, I must go down the street and pay seven dollars to the person who will inject me. I try to argue him into giving me the drug ahead of time. I want to know what the women use. But he thinks I do not want to pay the extra seven dollars. I offer to give him the twelve all at once, but he is confused and holds on to the injection. Finally, I leave.

I pass the Guadlupena one more time and note every detail—the neon sign jutting from the second story with the word *far-*

macia on the long leg of the L, Guadlupena on the short, and the right angle of the sign a cozy perch for a round-faced clock.

There are no perpendicular corners near the border, but you can't miss Sam's. It begins at a point and goes on to consume a triangular block. Inside is a big space with small square tables and many waiters, all anxious to pull out a chair for a *señorita*. I order a *piña colada* promptly and then set about selecting Mexican dishes. It is as complicated as a Chinese menu. The waiter helps to simplify matters by recommending a platter that has a little of everything. I accept his advice with excess gratitude.

By the time I leave Sam's, only the liquor stores have their lights on. I make my way down a dark alley past a crowd of shacks with tin corrugated roofs. I can just barely make out the letters of the large neon sign for El Rio Andy's. On reaching the bridge, I am directed to the booths on the right side for the return to the States. The small immigration office with its plastic bus-terminal chairs merges with the offices of the storefront *especialistas*. I hand the guard a dime.

"Wait. You get change. It's only two cents to cross back from Mexico," he says, handing me a nickel and three pennies before directing me to the immigration officer assigned to check purchases.

"You, American?" he asks. I nod and he motions me through without looking into my bag. It is sinking in—this border thing. All you need is two cents and Anglo skin.

On the bridge I take a last look at Reynosa. The cross of the old cathedral can be seen rising from the center of town. I pass by the grazing cows and the goats held by ropes attaching them at strange angles to the trees of the bank. On the American side, the saucer marquee of the Don José Plaza rotates high on a pedestal, advertising the specials of the day.

Steam is rising from the surface of the pool as the heated moisture hits the chilly air. The deserted patio looks sinister. In the lobby the retirees are taking bets on what will be the luncheon special.

Archer Park, across from the hotel, could be a village green with a coconut tree in place of a cannon. Four spokes of pavement radiate from a small wooden gazebo in the center of the manicured lawn. The park is empty, but around the perimeter cars are parked, each with a driver sitting idly. It takes a while before I see they are dealing dope.

On the other side of the park is the sole paper for McAllen's fifty thousand people—the *McAllen Monitor*—in a new one-story brick building. The printing presses click away behind the desks for reporters and the counter for classifieds.

The sounds of activity reassure me; small as it is, the newsroom looks like a serious place. I feel confident that her name is on record somewhere amidst the orderly noise. But I am uncertain whether to ask for help in finding it or to try to get it on my own.

"Don't tell them what you're doing until you're ready to leave town. Contracts out on people's lives." The warnings from the CDC team flash through my head. I am not worried about physical harm, only that it will be harder to get information if people know what I am up to. But I now have no choice. Without her name I cannot proceed.

Without stating why I want to look at them, I inquire about the location of back issues. October, I am told, is too recent for the microfilm but it should be with the pile organized month by month out on the counter.

If she died on the third, her obit should be in the paper a day or two later. I look at the fourth but it has nothing. Nor does the fifth. I go straight through to the sixteenth (except for Saturdays when no edition is printed). The thick Sunday edition is devoted largely to engagements. I plow through pages and pages of young women wearing proper prenuptial smiles. Reluctant to ask for help, I go back over every page of each day of the week following her death. Finally, I give in.

"Do you think you can help me?" I ask a young woman sitting at a desk. We chat for a few minutes. I tell her I'm a reporter from New York and learn that she has just come down herself from a colder climate where she was a photographer. "I've been given a local beat but not as a photographer. They don't have women taking pictures on this paper. They think it's too complicated for a woman to work a camera."

"Isn't it?"

The quip establishes rapport. I tell her I am trying to find out the name of the woman who died from an illegal abortion. "You know if the paper carried it?"

"Not a story, but an obit. I remember because there was a picture."

I light up at this unanticipated dividend. I tell her I've combed the obits for the two weeks following her death.

"Mexican-Americans don't have a sense of time. They could have sent it in much later," she comments, as we find ourselves exhausting the October pile. I ask her whether she is certain it was in.

"No question. I remember what she looked like. In fact, we got so many calls from all over the country I couldn't get my own work done," she says, glancing at her watch with digital numbers similar to the squared-off golden dots that alternate temperature and time for the drivers pulling up to the teller in the bank across from the *McAllen Monitor*.

"Let me speak to my boss. He may remember."

A pleasant-looking fellow with a mustache joins us. "Sure I remember. It was on the obituary page. No article. To tell the truth, we were surprised at the interest outside McAllen. It didn't even make it as a news story here."

Carefully, he goes through page 8 of Section A—the obituary page. He puts aside October 7, October 6, October 5. At October 4, he stops.

"Just as I remember. Right in the middle of the page," he says. I eye the ragged hole in the middle of the October 4 obituary page. "Let me check the back room. We may have another copy."

"Sorry, that's the only one," he says when he returns.

I hesitate to display my disappointment. "Is there any other paper that would have carried it? A Spanish paper in town?"

" 'Fraid this is it."

(There is no Spanish-language newspaper, although McAllen is 90 percent Mexican-American. The *Monitor,* at this writing, has one Spanish-speaking reporter on its editorial staff of seven.)

I thank the editor for his help and wave goodbye to the reporter sitting at her desk. "Mexican-Americans lack a sense of time," she had said. But the announcement of the death, a day later, was as precise as the time on her digital watch.

McAllen Public Library is a new and fairly well stocked place. Film showings are posted alongside notices of community events at the various Baptist churches in town. There is a magazine-reading room, a children's library, a record library, a typing room, and a room with a Xerox machine. Back issues of the *Monitor* are available, full sized or on microfilm. The back issues begin with January of 1978. The librarian says she will have to check about October of 1977.

"If you return in about a month, we should have it on microfilm. We're only up to August," she says apologetically.

I thank her and leave. Now what, I wonder.

It seems an unlikely place for the official highway green, but the sign is not official, just green. As soon as I read "La Piedad Cemetery," I come down hard on the brakes, back up the car, and point it in the direction of the arrow. I know it is right—one of those flashes commonly called intuitive. It is right because I am not expecting anything.

I follow the dirt path. There is a light mist in the air. The local TV weatherman refers to it as "running"; he explains, with many meteorological visual aids, what occurs when two wet currents traveling in opposite directions meet. "Similar to England," he notes, "except here we have the Gulf on one side and the ocean on the other." The weather report is eerie. That McAllen, a town caught in the crunch between two cultures, should also be trapped in the middle of opposing air currents has an unsettling metaphoric patness.

On both sides of the road is a neglected growth—a brownish brush that blends in with the muddy path. I travel slowly, the car hesitantly plowing through the fog. I am approaching a narrow stream; its small wooden crossing looks like a rotting pier long since abandoned by a bungalow owner. I look around. Not a single car, not a single person. I decide to check things out before taking the car over.

I am expecting stillness; instead, colors jump forward, as if aggressive imps are hidden somewhere. The only forms in motion that I can see are those of little boys; five heads, covered with thick dark hair, dart about as they pursue with a slingshot a bird in a tree.

CAMINO A SU DERECHA VELOCIDA 10 MPH reads a handmade sign painted with dark red clublike lines like clotting subway graffiti. An arrow points to the simple entrance gate; the name *La Piedad* accommodates the curve of the iron arch. I strain to read the official sign beyond: NO SE PERMITE INSTALACIONES DE CEMENTO O OTROS ARTEFACTOS QUE OBSTRUYAN O NO CON- TRIBUYAN AL MEJORAMIENTO DE ESTE CEMENTERIO. I can make out most of it. Not permitted, something of cement or other artifacts that destroy or do not contribute to the betterment of this cemetery. A sweet directive. I run back to the car with its righthand door still flung wide open. The crossing will support a car, even an audacious Olds, if I move slowly.

Once a friend and I walked around an old cemetery in Nantucket. It was early March, and we were determined to get some grave rubbings. Daffy and affected, we took pictures of each other lying dead with the oldest stones our headrests. The graveyard was a grim place, and the only way to respond to its morbidness was to go camp.

The weather is the same today as it was then, but La Piedad is vibrant with color: the orange red of fire, the aqua of water, the deep pink of sunsets, and the blood red of berries. The elemental colors are encompassed by a profusion of pastels unknown to my northern eye—pale lavenders, pale pinks, pale corals—hues of unpainted fingernails.

La Piedad is the only place in McAllen where nature has not been landscaped. It has a careless random design. The indigenous mesquite trees—wide-trunked and withery-branched with leaves that look soft enough to tickle—mingle with round short shrubs, tall trees that taper off like the quill of a pen, lush banana trees, and one large dead palm refusing to look decadent.

Close to the entrance, the graves fall into something approaching a pattern. Perhaps it would be more accurate to say they cluster, each group unofficially defined by a life-sized figure standing above—a Madonna waiting inside a blue scalloped tub. There are saints galore in robes so red they make suffering look royal. The mist mutes the aggressive piety of religious gestures.

The thin white arms of Jesus pinned to the white stone grave overlap the wire veins connecting the petals of the pale pink coronas. The effect is spookily ornate, like a standing lamp whose iron base turns into the claws of a bird.

La Piedad rotates, as the colorfully tiled tombstones depicting Biblical figures facing urgent sunsets spin the cemetery from Whitman sampler to Pre-Raphaelite painting before coming full circle into a commercial for heaven.

All the writing on the graves is in Spanish. The dead are named, dated, and *"recuerdo"* by *"esposos, madres,* and *hijos."* The family of R. L. Cruz uses black and white dime-sized tiles to honor his memory, making his grave marker a lasting game board. Standing nearby is the dark-skinned St. Martin, the only saint with short black hair. Were it not for their robes, the others— in long permed hair painted yellow—would resemble every denim-clad dude in town.

Toward the far end of the cemetery, the five little Mexican boys are still in pursuit of the bird. They carry on their chase amidst mounds of earth unnaturally tiny. Small pudgy females stand on short columns, one hand holding on to a small fold of stone fabric and a little leg slightly lifted with the knee bent, a cherub "holding it in" forever.

I read the nearest marker: *Santos Figuero, Julio 1, 1977, muerto Julio 3, 1977.* It is the babies' graveyard. The tiny mounds are tightly clustered, covered with a sheet of coronas.

I walk the other way toward the larger mounds and stop at a homemade grave. No tile; just a rusty peanut can placed atop a cement slab which someone started to paint aqua but never finished. The paint spills over, leaking down the six-inch slab in unruly squirts. A large applesauce jar has had its paint job similarly interrupted.

The cross at the head of the grave has never been started; it stands granite gray with two strands of black beads draped around it. The first strand rests around the center of the cross; the second, slung over at a diagonal, looks like a disco dancer's pocket purse.

In the distance is freshly dug dirt, too fresh to approach. The newly placed dead do not have markers, making them impossible to identify, and the rich-looking soil piled on high gives the impression someone is buried alive.

At the far end of the cemetery fewer trees grow. Two pieces of pipe double as a cross. A single plastic flower is sticking out from the vertical pipe. Missing are the miniature tile murals and the Biblical timetables announcing death as a departure point for eternity.

A few feet away lies the runway strip of the McAllen airport. A small plane is speeding toward take-off. It rushes by and in a few seconds disappears. Without realizing it, I have placed myself next to a grave that looks the right age. Neither brand-new nor old.

I hesitate to disturb the fragile easel supporting the Styrofoam cross. An aluminum grave marker is stuck in the earth like a meat thermometer. I look around to make sure no one is watching before pushing over a lavender twirl. On top of the marker are letters printed in black: CEBALLOS FUNERAL HOME. My heart begins to pound. The rest of the letters are cavities punched in the tin. I am certain the entire cross will topple if I press too hard. It's hard to make out the letters. It is easier to deal with numbers.

The year of birth appears to be 1950. I remove my mittens to get to the date I need—the day she died. Again, I push aside the twirl attached to the cross obstructing my view. I can now make it out. *October 3, 1977.* My hands are shaking. How many people in McAllen could have died on October 3, 1977, at the age of twenty-seven?

The imploring faces of the saints, the cherubic smiles of the angels, the outstretched arms of Jesus, the haunting passivity of the Virgin Mary, the planes taking off, the little boys with the slingshot shooting at the birds. All around are desperate emotions —escape, flight, pursuit. And finally, La Piedad, piety.

Twenty-seven years was not enough time. She came close. Right next to the speediest exit out of McAllen, Texas. That is where she lies. Rosaura Jimenez—that is her name.

I've never been comfortable with conversions, especially the kind by which a person becomes a symbol. With anxious appetites, we took hold of "the poor Chicana woman," ready to bury her in rhetoric.

What irony that she who lies dead from an illegal abortion should have been given the name that symbolizes "life"— Rosaura, a rose—to those who oppose abortion and demonstrate with live roses.

If there is to be a symbol, an icon, a rallying cry, a slogan, a saint, a martyr, let it not be the long-stemmed flower with petals of red. Or even the Virgin Mary in her aqua tub. Let it be a real woman—Rosaura Jimenez—who died in 1977 at the age of twenty-seven. Mexican-American; Mexican; American; it doesn't matter on which side of the border one is born, if one is a woman trying to walk the earth with dignity and pride.

TWO THE DOCTORS

Dr. Daniel Chester

Chester, Landrum, and Smith. It could be an old established law firm, slightly stuffy and always prudent, in the British tradition. But it is not. Chester, Landrum, and Smith are three doctors who practice obstetrics and gynecology. Although the pleasant new professional building resembles all the others clustered around McAllen General Hospital, it differs in one important respect: it is the only place where a woman can go to have a legal abortion.

I pick up a copy of *Newsweek* as I wait for my appointment. Dan Chester is my first important contact—someone who actually knew Rosaura, saw what she looked like, listened to the sound of her voice, watched her as she fought to stay alive and then as she begged to die in peace.

I have heard good things about Dr. Chester. He is the doctor who informed the public health officials of Rosaura's death. Otherwise, she might have been no more than an unpilfered obit in the *McAllen Monitor*.

Shortly after the Jimenez case, four other women—all poor, all Mexican-American—were hospitalized with unusual postabortion complications. Dr. Chester was concerned and felt it a duty to tell the federal authorities about the statistically unlikely quintet of cases.

Ordinarily, Dan Chester shuns publicity. It is not congruent with his image of a professional. But this was no ordinary occurrence, and Dan Chester agreed to go on "Good Morning America" to discuss it. A sense of duty compelled him to do so. He does not like to see young women die. To him, the seeking of an illegal abortion is not the crime; the crime is the fact that a woman has no other recourse.

No, you could not conclude that Rosaura crossed the border because she couldn't pay for a safe abortion, he told Americans as they sipped their morning coffee. Too simplistic. Mexican-American women might go over to Reynosa for a number of reasons. They have a fair amount of shame about sex as well as a need for privacy. Dan Chester respects privacy. When he was asked to speak at a memorial service held in Washington, D.C., for the "poor Chicana who died from an illegal abortion in Mexico after Medicaid money was cut off," he refused. Such a public display of mourning struck him as undignified.

"The doctor will see you now," says a middle-aged Anglo nurse, as the last patient leaves the office. "Follow me, please," she says as we pass the examining rooms with their sterilizers, stirrups, basins, mirrors, stainless-steel sinks, dilators, syringes, sterile gloves, jelly, and speculums looking like steely duck bills—all the equipment essential to enter and exit from a woman's insides with a minimum of mess.

"Just wait a minute, hon, the doctor will be out shortly."

In a few minutes a large-framed man with a light brown crew cut appears. Although he appears to be in his forties, Dan Chester looks as if he is trying out for a college fraternity. There is something both accommodating and ingenuous in his manner.

He knows why I am here; Frances Kissling of the National Abortion Federation has arranged the meeting on the phone. But he asks me to explain it once again, freshen up his memory if I don't mind. I tell him I am concerned with the issues of women's health and was drawn to the area by the report of the first Medicaid-related abortion death.

Dan Chester is astonished at how much interest the case has aroused around the country. "Down here in McAllen, hardly anyone seems to have taken note. Living so close to the border, we hear about deaths of one kind or another every day. I guess people around here are used to these things."

I ask him what made him decide to publicize the death. He mentions the four additional cases.

"We don't see that very often, so I thought I would let the authorities in on it. I also thought it important to let people know about the dangers in Reynosa. I appealed to a local TV person down here to do the story. He did, but he left out the crucial information and just concentrated on the sensational parts. After we saw the additional complications, they ran some spots on TV that warned women about the dangers of Mexican abortions. That was in October. At the end of this past January we had another cluster; this time three more infected abortion cases. Last week I saw a girl, mother of six children, thirty-three, separated, her youngest child age two, who showed up in the emergency room with fever and vaginal bleeding. All the girl would say is she fell."

"Why do you think the woman wished to conceal her abortion?"

"The girls are often afraid," he answers, using the vocabulary made comfortable by habit and training. Although I suspect Dan Chester is open to learning, this is not the appropriate moment. I move on to the question of what it is the women fear.

"Oh, fear of medical opinion, questions about legality. Many women are working here illegally, and the institutional setting is intimidating."

Dr. Chester is not so slow, after all! He has picked up on "women," and his answers indicate some insight into situations not of his own experience.

Silently, I reproach myself for judging him too quickly. It was wrong to assume he automatically projects his own values onto others.

"They all deny they have sought an abortion. Even when they come into the emergency room with profuse vaginal bleeding, they say they have had a fall. I guess they have all seen *Gone With the Wind,*" Dr. Chester says with a light tone. "They believe that a fall can cause a miscarriage."

I return to the subject of the fear and intimidation aroused by institutional settings.

His answer is circumspect; he concedes that such factors are possible influences, but he is not comfortable tying close events together; links between behavior and motivation are best left loose. He looks relaxed as he places his large hands behind his head which he tilts back.

"Let me give you a little background about this part of the country," he says after he gives his body a good stretch. "There has been a fantastic change in the people growing up on this side. Several thousand homes in Brownsville, just a short distance away, have no plumbing. Still, the people living in them are much better off than they are in Mexico. Do you know that Mexico is the fastest growing nation in the Western Hemisphere? By the year 2000, the population will equal that of the United States. And each week one thousand Mexicans enter this country."

Dr. Chester likes figures; he is comfortable with the concrete. I can imagine him in his spare time reading books of lists. "The Mexican government has been encouraging large families, but now is quietly starting family planning," Dr. Chester confides, lowering his voice as if he is letting me in on a secret. "The Latin Americans who grow up here want birth control and sterilization. Ninety-five percent of the abortions I do are on Latin American women."

After finding out that he performs about twenty a month, I multiply that figure by two hundred dollars—the rough profit from a two-hundred-and-thirty-dollar, routine first-trimester abortion. Using the figure supplied by the CDC, I compute that Dr. Chester takes in about four thousand dollars a month from abortion—close to fifty thousand dollars a year for work that takes about five hours a week.

While I assume that, like other gynecologists, Dr. Chester earns at least one hundred thousand dollars annually, he does not place himself among the rich. In the land of the King Ranch and oil refineries, where a rig is as common as a tractor, Dr. Chester is a man of comfortable, but modest, means. On the scale of Texas wealth, he would not rank high. He must work to earn his money; in fact, this afternoon is the only day besides Sunday that he does not attend patients. Aware he has made an exception to see me before he goes home to change into his tennis clothes, I am anxious to move along.

"How comfortable are the women in discussing their sexuality?" I ask, explaining that many people have suggested that the Mexican-American woman, filled with great shame about her body, seeks abortions across the border primarily for privacy, not money.

"How comfortable?" Dr. Chester repeats, bringing his hands down from behind his neck and placing them squarely on the glass top of his desk. "Well, let me see. If a woman is a lesbian, and we do have some, you know, or if she wants to talk about a beard scratching her vagina, well . . ." and here Dr. Chester takes a deep breath, "I don't imagine she comes to me. I just don't know enough, to be perfectly truthful, and she probably wouldn't feel comfortable."

"Fair enough. Whom does she go to?"

"I have a younger partner who she would probably prefer," Dr. Chester says with a candor I find endearing.

I ask him whether he finds much difference between the Chicana women and American women.

"Educated Latin girls are just like other girls, I would say. They are all career oriented. The second generation of rich Mexican men, the sons of fathers who always had girlfriends on the side, are having a new experience. The younger girls they meet won't put up with it," Dr. Chester says approvingly. "You can just see from the columns of divorces in the paper. Women in their twenties and thirties don't want to be used."

I ask Dr. Chester if the expression *"me uso,"* employed by a Mexican-American doctor I interviewed, is a common way to describe intercourse.

"Yes, that is the expression, but the attitudes are different. I'll give you an example. I did a hysterectomy on an older woman. The first thing she wanted to know is if it is okay to tell her husband she can no longer have sex with him. Yet her daughter wants to know just the opposite, 'When can I start again.' I think the ethnic background is less important than education."

Again I refer to my interview with the Mexican-American doctor. "While agreeing that education is key, he speaks with pride of his plans to make his son into a rooster by taking him to a prostitute across the border at age fifteen while his daughters remain 'clean little chicks' here in McAllen."

"He does, does he," Dr. Chester says, breaking into a roar and shaking his head back so far it looks as though he might topple over. "My goodness. Well, you see, I am a Methodist, and my sexual experience has been only with my wife. I was a virgin when we married and have never known anyone else. When I was in the Army, I used to go to a nearby brothel. I can still remember talking with the girls at night. There was little else to do and they were real friendly. Some of them I found quite interesting to talk to. But when I was finished talking, I would go home to bed."

Dr. Chester pauses for a moment as he looks at a photograph of his three daughters. "Golly, time does pass by. I remember when I first moved to McAllen eleven years ago. It was a real small town then, but it is growing very rapidly. There is more opportunity here than in any other part of Texas right now. I'm not sure I'll like it if it gets much bigger."

Dr. Chester assumes a pensive air, and I realize we have gotten far away from the original matter.

"I know this is your afternoon off, and I don't want to keep you too long," I say, ready to veer us back on course. "Perhaps you could review exactly what happened to the woman who died. Before going into the medical details, I'm curious about your impressions of her as a person. What do you know about her life?"

"Well, they say she was a housekeeper for a white man, but I have no proof of that," Dr. Chester quickly adds. "She has a cousin who works in the hospital as an orderly. You might contact him for that kind of information. He was the one who told us she had an abortion. He gave us that information voluntarily."

I ask Dr. Chester to go over the medical story for me.

"When I was first called to the hospital, she was already very ill," he says as he takes a deep breath.

"I suspected right away that she had an abortion, although she kept on denying it. She came in yellowish green and shaking. It took us a while to diagnose her. Finally, we pinned it down to an infection called *Clostridium perfringens.*"

I ask Dr. Chester to spell it out for me.

"I think this is right," he says, staring at the words he has written in my pad. "It's not at all common," he says, as if to explain his uncertainty.

"It's an organism that is present in dirt, feces, and can come out of the intestinal tract. It is the same family as tetanus, except she would have done better with tetanus itself. We had another complication with tetanus following an abortion, and she survived. At best, there's only a ten percent chance of survival with what she had.

"I even told her she might not pull through. I hoped that would free her to talk."

"Did it?"

"Not for the first several days."

"How long was she in the hospital?"

"Eight days, I believe."

"And what was the course of her illness?"

"This particular microorganism produces a variety of toxins. One breaks down the red blood cells." As Dr. Chester speaks, I remember the most vivid detail—the blood coming from her eyes. "The debris from the red blood cells had accumulated in the filtering mechanism of her kidney. There were other toxins that are harmful to different systems. The muscle cells of her heart and the liver and the immunization systems were all adversely affected.

"First we performed a tracheotomy on her to help her with her breathing. And then we decided to do a hysterectomy, even though we felt great reluctance to remove a woman's childbearing organs when she is so young."

"Even when she is so sick?"

"Well, that is the point. I did not think she would live, so it didn't seem appropriate to worry about future children. She had such massive pelvic infection that we were left with very little choice. And we weren't certain of the source. We had her on dialysis; she had tracheal tubing in her, and she was in intensive care the whole time. Considering that she had what you might call generalized organ failure, she hung on pretty long.

"She was still denying she had the abortion even toward the end. Since she could not talk because of the tracheotomy, I asked her to squeeze once if she had the abortion, and twice if she didn't. She kept on squeezing twice. Then, I'll be darned, she changed her mind. Finally, she did squeeze once. Beats me to this day as to why she decided to give in."

I do not ask Dr. Chester why he kept pressing, since her cousin, the orderly, had already told him she had the abortion, and instead I inquire at what point she finally decided to "give in."

"Six hours before she died."

"Was she alone?"

"No. Her family was there and her friends visited. One woman, in particular, was very attentive. She kept on massaging her legs throughout."

"How did the family react?"

"They didn't do anything to me. Sometimes when a woman dies in childbirth, the family threatens to kill the doctor. But nothing of that sort happened. She came and went and would have been forgotten were it not for the national publicity."

"What I would like to know is how do you think this sort of thing can be prevented from happening in the future?"

"Now that, I would say, is a real interesting question. I've never thought about it before. Give me a minute or two."

I watch Dr. Chester. I am no longer asking questions that involve description—what took place; how did she look; what was written down on the hospital chart; how do you spell it; what was done to save the woman's childbearing organs, and failing that, the woman herself. Dr. Chester has sounded relatively free of bias; he seems humane, liberal, even if a bit naive. He is still puzzling over the question of prevention. His brow is furrowed.

"A problem pregnancy is a medical problem, as far as I'm concerned," he starts out, "and no medical problem should be excluded from Medicaid.

"There should be a way to treat a woman without money.

Theoretically, such a woman could exist." I do not want to interrupt his flow to question the emphatic "theoretically." "And what's more, an abortion death is different from, let's say for the purposes of argument, a cardiac death."

Good, I think, silently cheering Dr. Chester on to the conclusion of his logic.

"So, I would say," he continues, his Southern drawl noticeable for the first time, "that in cases like this," and again Dr. Chester pauses, "in cases like this, the death can be prevented."

"How so?"

"A woman can always say no."

Noting my startled expression, he adds, "I don't think you can use intercourse as a vehicle for marriage."

"How do you know Rosaura Jimenez was doing that?"

"I don't. It's just that there are a lot of drugs around; it's a border town, lots of marijuana, loose respect for parents. It all goes together in my mind. No, don't get me wrong. I'm not perfect myself; I'm human, too. I was on a plane and I picked up a copy of *The Happy Hooker.* Well, I'm going to tell you the gosh honest truth. There was a point on that plane when I had to stop reading."

As I prepare to leave, Dr. Chester says, "It's been a pleasure talking to someone who understands scientific thinking."

Dr. Raphael Garza

Right across from McAllen General Hospital, on the outside of a new one-story professional building (not unlike Dan Chester's), a fancy script spells out the name Raphael Garza, followed by the letters *M.D.* and the medical symbol.

I do not have an appointment and walk in off the street. The office is crowded with term-swollen women who eye an Anglo with suspicion. The receptionist is enclosed in a booth, like a bank teller. There is a small hole for speaking, but the woman behind the glass is checking over a medical chart.

As I stand waiting for her attention, I notice a plaque on the door to the doctors' offices (Raphael Garza is in practice with two other doctors.): ALL LABORATORY X-RAYS AND CANCER STUDIES CHARGES WILL BE CASH. THANK YOU.

Below the plaque is a handwritten sign:

> Welfare Patients, effective January 1st, 1977: 1. you must have monthly card on every visit 2. you must sign for every visit 3. you must pay cash if you don't have your welfare card 4. you must pay for any non-covered services.

The last two commands are underlined.

A duplicate of the sign is in the waiting room. Pretending to be an anxious patient sizing up the number ahead of me, I scan the room, trying to memorize a line from the sign before scribbling it down when no one is looking. But everyone is looking. Looking hard. And I put my notebook away.

"Miss, can I help you?" asks a voice through the small opening.

"I'd like to make an appointment to see the doctor."

"Have you ever been here before?" the receptionist asks, sensing it is unlikely.

"No. I'm not a patient. It's a business call." And then, noting her puzzled look, I add, "I've just come from Dr. Chester's," making my request more confusing but impossible to ignore. I see the list of patients' names extending through the afternoon on the appointment book. At least the doctor is in.

"When is his last appointment?" I ask, as she continues to stall.

"Let me go inside and talk to him," she says, uncertain about how to handle me.

"Fine," I respond, taking out my notebook as soon as she disappears. The women waiting watch me copy down the sign. They probably think I am with some social agency checking up on them, contemplating adding further financial requirements and safeguards. I cannot correct their impression.

"The doctor will see you now," the receptionist announces.

I am surprised but do not insist on waiting. Inside the empty office is a picture of a middle-aged man with a mustache that stiffens out to a thin curl. Next to him stands a woman, fully corseted and finely coiffed, surrounded by several children, all posed in front of a large house. Alongside the medical texts on the shelves are several busts of Madonnas and saints, lined up in their plaster-of-paris robes like trophies won at a carnival stand. I take a seat facing the desk. LET'S COMPROMISE. WE'LL DO IT MY WAY, reads a small plaque.

"My girl tells me you are here on business, that you have just come from Dr. Chester's. What can I do for you? I am in the middle of an examination, so I have only a few minutes," the doctor says when he walks in.

Raphael Garza has the smoothness of a man who receives pedicures with regularity. His fingernails are polished, his hair sprayed, and his pants, extending beneath his starched white medical coat, have a crease that looks sharp enough to cut. The diamond pinky ring, the thinly pointed shoes, the fancy wrist band seem designed to complement the plaster saints and afford a balance between the material world and that of the spirit.

Dr. Garza wants to know how I got to his office.

The name of the only Anglo ob-gyn office nearby was an effective passport with the receptionist and I use it again.

"I know Dr. Chester," he says. "What were you doing there?"

"Checking into the death of Rosaura Jimenez, the woman who died from an illegal abortion. Did you know her?"

"Hortensia," he calls out, "go get me the Jimenez file."

The receptionist brings in a chart and Dr. Garza, lowering his dark-rimmed glasses, looks it over. "Yes, she was a patient of mine in July 1973. It says here that I delivered her baby."

I am surprised. I had no idea he treated her. I merely thought that, as a Mexican-American doctor, he might know of her or her relatives. "Tell me a bit about her."

"That is not possible. I have the largest practice in town. I cannot remember them all," he says impatiently. "No one could who delivers as many babies as I do," he adds defensively.

"You are an obstetrician?"

"No, a family doctor. But I deliver more babies than anyone else in town. I have been delivering babies here in McAllen for twenty years. I started out with a small maternity clinic. I still have it behind the office building. That is where I do my uncomplicated births."

Dr. Garza performs between seventy and one hundred deliveries a month. He also mentions that he is a backup for *parteras*. I have never heard the term before. He explains that they are midwives, old Mexican women who deliver babies for those who don't want a doctor. I ask if it is legal for the midwives to perform abortions.

"To me, all abortions are illegal," he says brusquely. "I call them criminal abortions whether they are legal or not."

When I point out that women seek them no matter what they are called, he shrugs indifferently. "Yes, all the girls have to do is cross the border. Usually they go with a friend. A nonmedico, maybe a pharmacist or nurse, freezes a Foley catheter prior to inserting it into the woman's cervix.

"The catheter is a long, hollow rubber tube a quarter- to a half-inch in diameter. Frozen, it can be inserted easily; as it defrosts, the cervix dilates a bit. Uterine contractions follow, eventually causing a 'spontaneous abortion.' Of course, it is a rather primitive and dangerous technique. Infection is common, and the uterus can easily be perforated."

I ask Dr. Garza why he thinks the women cross the border when they can get a safe abortion at Dr. Chester's.

"Let me see how I can explain it to you. I'll put it this way," he says, sizing me up first. "If a man wishes to fool around, see another woman, he would seek out privacy. It makes sense, no?"

Ignoring his question, I ask about money.

"They have the money or they can get it. This is a rich place."

"What about the signs in your office concerning welfare and Medicaid cards?"

"That is what I mean. The government pays for that when the

girls can't. And when the government doesn't, they have ways of rounding up the money. That is why we have the signs. They can't fool us. They will sell their rosary beads if they want something badly enough. If they want their baby delivered in good hands, they find the money some way. I've seen it myself," Dr. Garza states conclusively.

"Getting back to Rosaura Jimenez. Did you or your partners treat her in the hospital?"

"Not that I know of. But we see so many. Let me check it for you." He dials a number. "Record room, Dr. Garza speaking," he says into the beige receiver. And then turning to me, "I don't think we had anything to do with her. Damn, I was just disconnected. Hortensia, come here. Try getting me the record room and as soon as you do, buzz me on three."

"I have it," he calls out when the phone is buzzed. "Dr. Garza over here. I want the chart of Jimenez. First name?" he asks, turning toward me.

"Rosaura."

I jot down the chart number repeated aloud by Dr. Garza.

"And the date of admission? September twenty-sixth. Date of death? October third. Good. And who is the admitting doctor on the record? Howard Hughes. Thank you. That's all.

"I didn't think we had anything to do with the case, but we take turns in the emergency room, so it is always good to check."

"Where is Dr. Hughes?"

"He's in practice with Dr. Rivas, a few blocks away."

"Fine. Maybe he will be able to give me more information. Thank you for your time."

As Dr. Garza rises to shake my hand, I can smell his after-shave lotion. The odor lingers with me in the waiting room, where I stand openly copying down the signs about payment. The women, who had been staring at the blank wall of the waiting room, again stare at me.

Dr. Homero Rivas

I enter the office of Howard Hughes without an appointment. By now I know the routine. I'm here to see the doctor. No, I am not a patient. I'm here on business. I've just spoken with Dr. Garza, I say, using the last visit as a passport to the next. The receptionist seems uncomfortable.

"Dr. Hughes isn't coming in this afternoon," she says after hesitating.

I tell her I will speak with one of his associates.

She takes my name and puts it down at the end of a long list. I ask her how much time she anticipates the wait will be. About two or three hours, she says.

At 5:30, I enter the office of Dr. Homero Rivas. I do not see a single cross; there are no kitschy sayings; nor is there a picture of a smiling family. In their stead are photographs, framed in lucite, of a long-haired man, backpacking. He appears to be in his mid-thirties. For the first time, I feel at home.

Homero Rivas is a short, wiry man with dark black hair. Instead of being oiled back in the style of Dr. Garza, Rivas's hangs over his ears, overlapping the frames of his aviator glasses. His manner is informal yet he never stands still. Immediately we are on a first-name basis. "But not Homero; it's Homer."

Homer looks pleased when I ask if he is a storyteller. "Most of the doctors here haven't even read Homer. You're not from down here, are you?"

"I am from New York City."

"I could tell. You know something? They all think they are so smart in New York. I got some of my training there, and I can honestly say that I practice better medicine down here than what I saw up there. Doctors there are cold and calloused. Of course, they're smart, like all Jews. But they have no feeling for their patients. You're not Jewish by any chance, are you?"

"Yes, I am."

"That makes two of us. I am from the oldest and the most

aristocratic of the Jews, the ones who once lived in Spain and then settled in Mexico. I was raised in the tradition of the Jewish intellectual. That is why I could see through all those doctors in New York, the ones who deny their Jewishness. And when you come right down to it, they are not really intellectual. They drop a lot of names—culture, the arts, and stuff like that—but they're totally square and totally materialistic. They could never accept me. I came back here to the border to be with my people. I had long hair and wore blue jeans and sandals. I lived in a little house that had a garden full of weeds. One day a woman in a Cadillac drives up and asks, 'How much do you charge for gardening?' And I answer, 'The owner of the garden lets me sleep with her and I don't charge her anything.' And do you know what? She believes every word. So you see, that is how someone like myself is viewed."

I do not trust him. He is too anxious to appear hip. "What about Rosaura Jimenez?" I ask, abruptly.

"Dr. Hughes admitted her to the hospital. But I was her real doctor. I'm the one who knew Rosie."

"Rosie?"

"Yes. She liked Rosie. Not Rosaura."

"Like Homer instead of Homero."

"Everyone down here wants to sound Anglo. I have taken it one step further. Remember, it's not the English who founded Western civilization. It's the Greeks."

I want to tell Homer pomposity is not hip. Instead I tell him he is the first person I've met who actually knew her. "Dr. Chester treated her when she was dying, but he had little to say about her except he thought she was a maid to an Anglo."

"That just shows how much he knows."

"In all fairness, he wasn't sure."

"Nah, Dan Chester never gets to know his patients the way I do."

"When can we get together to talk?"

Homer has to judge a beauty contest in Mission at 7:00, but he is free any time afterward. We agree that he will come to the La Posada at about 10:00 to discuss Rosaura.

"No, Rosie," he reminds me as I wave goodbye.

Despite some personal reservations about Homer, I feel elated. This is the break I have been waiting for.

At 11:00 I call the hospital where Homer is on call. I wait for the operator to have him paged. "Sorry, miss, he doesn't answer." An emergency must have held him up, I conclude. I ask her for a number where he can be reached. "Just a minute, please, I'll check that for you." I am struck by how easy it is to obtain information in McAllen; not once has the operator asked who I am. "Sorry, Dr. Rivas has left no number," she reports. I try his service. "No, he has not checked in all night. I'm not expecting to hear from him, but if you'd like to leave your name, I'll give it to him as soon as he phones in. Probably tomorrow. He's on call at the hospital. You might try to reach him there." I hang up and dial his office, but nobody picks up.

It is 11:30 and I've exhausted the TV programing; all that remains are the UPI wires. I watch as words about a riot in South Africa are telegraphed to the accompaniment of Muzak, which, at fifteen-minute intervals, is interrupted by a detailed weather forecast.

I try the hospital again. Nothing has changed; Homer cannot be reached. Lucky I'm not hemorrhaging to death, I think to myself, as I decide what to do next.

I remember Homer's boast that he is one of the few doctors who is willing to list his home number in the telephone book. The others don't want to risk being bothered by patients. Not me, he had said. While I wait for the phone to ring, I flip to Chester. I see nothing in his name, but there is a Chester with a woman's name. Dan has used an old medical ploy—his wife's name—to ensure that patients won't disturb him.

"No, don't go to sleep. I'm on my way over. I'll be there in less than five minutes," Homer assures me when I reach him at home.

"When do *you* sleep?" I ask when he arrives.

"Sleep? I need very little."

"You are a regular hyperactive child. Just like a New York

doctor," I chide him, as I take a seat on the floor. "Jogging, tennis, squash, surgery."

"No, I don't do those things. I climb mountains and raise horses. Did you see the trophy in my office for the Cayetaño Berrera?"

I remind Homer it's late.

"Late?"

"Late for me. Let's spend some time talking about Rosie."

"There is very little to say. You can't solve economic problems medically."

"Well, that is something to say. You are the first doctor I have spoken with who even acknowledges there is such a thing as an economic problem," I say, quoting Chester's "theoretical" poor woman.

"Oh, Chester. What can you expect? He is one of the most conservative doctors in town. We serve on many boards together, and he always votes in a reactionary way."

I point out, slightly defensively, that at least Chester is willing to do abortions; that next to a man like Garza, Chester comes out radical.

"To be an abortionist is not to be radical. I am radical, but I am not an abortionist.

"Of course I am in favor of abortions," Homer immediately adds. "That goes without saying. And I also think a woman should be free to have contraception. I don't even ask her if she is married when she comes to me for help with the pill or something like that. But I am still not an abortionist. It is a lowly thing to be, medically speaking. I don't think any doctor who takes himself seriously, and who really knows medicine, finds doing an abortion a challenge."

Were it not so late, I might be tempted to ask why doctors think practicing medicine is like scaling Mount Everest. But I want to move on. "When was the last time you saw Rosie?"

"I saw Rosie in the hospital. Even though she was very close to death, she raised her eyes when I called her name. I felt angry seeing her that way because I cared. I wondered why she couldn't tell me."

But I remind Homer that, according to the story that went out at the time of her death, she did tell her family doctor, and he in turn told her she would not be able to obtain a Medicaid abortion. "Weren't you her family doctor? Didn't you treat her before she had the abortion in Mexico?"

Homer looks uncomfortable. "I don't know what story you're referring to," he says irritably. "Lots of things were said when she died."

"Well, were you treating her or not?"

"Rosie came to me sometime in September with pains in her chest, and I gave her two shots for her condition."

"Which was?"

"Osteochondritis."

"Did she have any other symptoms?"

"Oh, she said something about missing her period."

"And what did you do?"

"You know something," Homer says, suddenly getting up from a chair and jumping on one of the double beds as if it were a trampoline, "I really don't feel like discussing this anymore. I am tired of it."

I consent to stop as soon as we run through a few more questions. "What kind of shots did Rosie get in Reynosa?"

"How should I know?"

"I just figured you were up on things, but I guess I was wrong."

Homer responds predictably. "Of course I know. They usually give them a shot of Depo-Provera to bring on the period. It won't work if the woman is pregnant, only if she is late. I'll tell you this much, many women are totally misinformed. They believe that they are getting an abortion when they get a shot. They don't understand their bodies."

"Did Rosie?"

"Rosie was a very smart girl, but I don't want to talk about her. You see this?" Homer asks as he gets up from the bed and joins me on the floor. "I made this vest," he says, unlooping a hook around a miniature carved tusk of ivory.

"The hook too?"

"I made the whole thing. Look at the inside." Homer opens

his vest so I can see the intricate embroidery on the silk lining. "Do you like it?"

"It's lovely."

"Here, have a feel."

"Homer, clearly you have an eye for the visual. Tell me what Rosie looked like."

"Very attractive, real petite."

"Homer, what is the name of the cousin of Rosie's who works as an orderly at the hospital?"

"I can't remember."

"What about the name of another relative."

"I don't know any."

"Some doctor you are!"

"I only knew her father," Homer says, sitting up. "He was a butcher, and he used to purchase his meat from my father's supermarket."

"Your father works in a supermarket?"

"No. He owns a whole chain. Haven't you seen them? They're all over. Rivas Markets. They cater to the Mexican community. We take food stamps even for beer and cigarettes and give credit. We're not like the others which are owned by Americans," Homer says, getting up from the floor as if ready to go.

"Well, what is the name of her father?"

"Look, I'm tired of this."

"Homer, the name of her father," I say without moving.

"I can't remember."

"Okay, then let's go back to the orderly. Or anyone who knew her. Anyone except a doctor," I add, as my own irritation begins to show.

"I don't think Rosie would like that. Anyway, what's in it for me?"

"Homer, I made an appointment with you to talk about a woman who died, a woman you expressed some concern about earlier. Remember?"

"Yeah, yeah, yeah. All the talk in the world isn't going to bring her back."

"Look, are you willing to talk or not? All I am asking for is the name of her cousin."

"You'll have to call my office in the morning."

"Homer, it *is* morning. It's ten to four."

Homer seems amused by my firm tone. "What do you want me to talk about?"

"I want you to leave."

"Come on, that's not fair. Give me another chance."

"Homer, you're acting like a brat. You may not need sleep, but I do," I say, getting up to hold open the door.

Persuaded that I am serious, Homer slowly gets ready to leave. Before stepping out the door, he stands in front of the mirror and watches himself carefully put the loop around the ivory tusk of his vest.

As soon as I close the door I reach for the telephone and get the number of Texas International. I must cancel my morning flight back. I still don't have anything to go on. After letting the phone ring for ten minutes, I get a response. With my flight canceled, I climb into bed, hoping to get some sleep before making a final attempt. The meeting with Homer has made it clear that I am on the wrong path. I must get away from doctors.

THREE **THE COUNSELORS**

Lila Burns

"There's a very low abortion rate in this area. Our people are very moral," Lila Burns, executive director of the local Planned Parenthood office, says softly as she sips a cup of coffee in the hotel's informal eatery. "When a woman gets pregnant down here, she gets married."

Lila Burns is an attractive woman dressed in a Givenchy tennis top. "My husband knows a lot of what is going on. He owns an automobile showroom along Route Twenty-three, the road to Reynosa. Most of the car places are drug fronts. That's where the kids get their sniffers for school. They found that out in a survey of the ninth grade. They're going to get a dog that can smell the drugs, one trained for that purpose."

I return to the problem of abortion, but Lila Burns does not see it as a problem. Pregnant women, she says, get married. Of the 6,500 patients who pass through Planned Parenthood, about 90 percent are married, she tells me, as if to document her assertion.

I ask her about the 650 who aren't married. What do they do?

"Have the babies," she says, without hesitation. "Just like the married ones." And then as an afterthought, she adds, "We do offer a vasectomy program for the men. But only five took advantage of it even though it's free."

I tell Lila Burns that up North vasectomy is popular with

working-class men. They can fool around more easily without having to worry about a woman who is not their wife becoming pregnant.

"No, it's different down here. It's very conservative. Seventy-five percent of the community is Catholic, and there is an active right-to-life movement. The men call up our clinic to check. 'Is my wife a patient?' they want to know. Sometimes I think it is better. We have a very low VD rate here. Almost nonexistent."

I am sure Lila Burns is telling the truth. However, there is no place in the country that has a nonexistent VD rate among its sexually active youth. But I let the matter pass. I want to discuss Rosaura Jimenez.

"Who does do the abortions for those women who want them? The woman who died surely wanted one."

"Well, *we* don't do abortions. We do refer the women, but we don't want them all coming to us; we can't take care of them all. We also don't actively recruit the young. But there are four M.D.'s who share an office suite in McAllen. They do it there. The Church is very dominant, you know. You can have an abortion on Saturday, but you must go to confession on Sunday. I have an assistant who got all flushed because the priest asked her where she worked. All she could answer is, 'I counsel people.' But it is all for the better. Because when they stopped the federal funding for abortion, only the affluent kids could get them. After that, we didn't have money for poor women, only for 'special cases.' I personally would have a hard time saying, 'You can't have an abortion. You're not a special case.' But my assistant has no problem that way."

The waiter asks us if we want more coffee. Lila Burns looks at me to see if I will have some before accepting.

"Most doctors here are very antiabortion," she whispers, with regret.

Lila Burns seems eager to come out well, as if she were being interviewed for a talk show. She demonstrates a demure concern. But it is as if some response were missing—the one that makes connections. I am meeting with her to discuss the abortion death of a twenty-seven-year-old woman.

The people who oppose abortions are her neighbors; they live in the fancy houses next to hers; they buy their cars from her husband; they are nice people. So is she.

"A lot of Mexican-American women come here to have their babies. They want the American citizenship. It costs them about two hundred dollars. There is a nurse-midwife, Sister Ann, you might talk to. She delivers many of their babies."

I ask Lila Burns whether the women know about public services.

"They know about food stamps. But they don't know about Medicaid abortions. We had a patient who came in for a pregnancy test and was going to Mexico for an abortion. Her cousin said, 'This is where you go.' You see, all the medical offices are open on Sunday and it's cheap there. That's where they're used to going; it's part of the shopping and socializing. They prefer to do it in Mexico."

"You mean Rosaura Jimenez would have preferred to get an abortion in Mexico over a safe one here if a safe one had been available."

"Yes. They want privacy. And it feels more like home. There is a pharmacy, the Guadlupena, where they all go for illicit drugs and abortions. That's where the woman who died went.

"She was living with her family. Her father is a pusher in Houston. She was a patient of Planned Parenthood, but she didn't come here. I know she was on the pill and going to college. She was due to graduate from Pan American University. Her parents didn't know about it."

It strikes me as unlikely that a college student who was a patient of Planned Parenthood would choose an illegal abortion over a safe one. I ask Lila Burns if she sees the discrepancy.

She concedes that it is unusual for a single woman—especially a Mexican-American—to come to Planned Parenthood on her own. "We don't see many. Most pregnant women seeking help have the baby. The poor have nothing else to do. They like it. Even the younger women wind up having the babies. Sometimes they give the baby to their mothers or aunts to bring up. It's quite typical to hear a woman say, 'I had one child and I gave it to my sister who couldn't have any,' or 'I have to go to a funeral today. My cousin's cousin died.' It's one big—how do you say . . . ?"

"Extended family?"

"Yes, that's the phrase I am looking for. The extended family works for the poor. They have hard lives here. This county, Hidalgo, has the lowest per-capita income in the U.S."

Lila Burns, pert as a doctor's receptionist, has a blurry soul. Somewhere she knows that something is wrong, but it is hard to pinpoint. It keeps on shifting, eluding her. No one is really bad. McAllen is a decent town.

"As I said, we don't actually perform abortions, but last year we did refer a hundred women to a group of doctors in Harlingen who are willing to take special cases."

I make note that Planned Parenthood accepted one hundred "special cases" for the entire year in the county with the lowest per-capita income in the United States.

Lila Burns, sensing my disapproval, adds that a special case has to pay only $130.00 instead of the full fee of $200.00.

"What about the woman who can't afford the one hundred and thirty?"

"Fortunately, we don't see many of them. Most don't want abortions. Recently a thirteen-year-old girl came to us. She became pregnant by a twenty-two-year-old man. Her mother wanted her to have the abortion, but the daughter wanted to have the child. You see what I mean," Lila Burns says with a touch of despair, as she butters a roll. Lila Burns may have the perennially sweet face of a receptionist, but like a president's wife, her sweetness covers a no-nonsense personality. She has her values, her concerns. She can see that it is unfortunate that a young woman cannot learn from her mother. After all, she has a daughter of her own. She hopes her daughter will "know better" when the time comes, she confides, without saying what it is she will "know better."

"I can't understand why people act against their own interests. I guess that is all they have to do—have babies."

Lila Burns genuinely regrets the diminished lives she witnesses, but she doesn't see how she contributes to them by accepting poverty as some congenital defect for which there is no corrective surgery. She believes in abortions for the young and the poor, and she is glad a few doctors are willing to do them. But she cannot get beyond gratitude. Outrage would be an indecent emotion— outrage that the doctors demand cash ahead of time, with no exceptions, and that the government virtually subsidizes their private practices by refusing to support facilities that charge less.

"The children of the poor grow up in crowded quarters, often no more than two rooms. They see sex at an early age. The problem is they still are ignorant of the biology even when they themselves come of age."

"How do most women feel about sex?"

Lila laughs quietly. "Oh, it's a wifely duty, not an enjoyed duty. The women are taught to satisfy their husbands. 'Last night when my husband used me' is how they put it. *'Me uso'* is the expression for sex," Lila remarks casually. "All the *cantinas* have 'ladies' for pleasure. Sex with the wife is just a release for the man.

"The women don't like it. When a doctor tells them they have an infection, the first thing they ask is, 'Is this a reason for my husband not to use me.' And they get very excited at the possibility."

Excited at the possibility of not having sex sounds like a joke. Excited at the possibility of not being used does not.

"Generally, the women are not in good condition. Two-thirds of the Pap smears show some kind of infection. Part of that is because it is a warm humid climate and the men are uncircumsized. There is a lot of cervicitis. But the women don't complain. They consider it normal. In fact, a suspect Pap test—a Class Two smear—is considered normal down here."

Lila Burns and I chat some more before she gives me the names of doctors to see, clinics to visit. She is going out of her way to be helpful. It is clear she does not want another abortion death. There is a feeling that if we talk about it but remain polite, it will go away.

Back in my room, I make a list of all the names Lila Burns has given me. In one instance, a sociology professor, she did not have the phone number but was pretty certain he is listed. She is right.

I make note of his number, and then, out of idle curiosity, I flip to "J," just to see how many Jimenezes there are in McAllen. If all else fails, I can call each number. Odds are that one is bound to be related to Rosaura.

There are fewer than I thought. Estela, Evangelina, Isabel, Jorge, Juan, Lucio, Moises, Oscar, Otela, Raymond, Rodrigor, and. . . . I do not go on to the last two names but pick up the phone and dial 9 for an outside line. As I wait for the tone, I stare at the name to make sure I am not imagining it. I am not; it's right there in black and white—Rosaura Jimenez. Suppose someone answers. What will I say? The phone rings. But nobody answers.

Daffodil, Date Palm, Jonquil, Jasmine, Ebony, Esperanza, Gumwood, Hackberry, Pecan, Sycamore, Shasta, Tamarack, Upas, Violet, Walnut, Wisteria. The streets cry out the names of flowers and trees, calling forth a jumpy fecundity, but the quiet new development betrays the nomenclature. There are neither trees nor fragrances, not even people, except for an occasional youth running alongside the road in a bright blue suit with chalk-white trim. The neat houses with their single boxwood shrubs look like they come from a catalogue.

Gardenia passes by, and I slow down. At the very end of Hibiscus is the number I am looking for—the number listed next to the name in the phone book.

I wonder if it ever occurred to the CDC to look there for Rosaura's address and phone number, to drive by her house and see how she lived. Perhaps, to knock on a neighbor's door and simply ask for information on the life of a woman desperate enough to seek an illegal abortion.

Rosaura's apartment could be any one of four units in the attached brick garden complex. One has a garden chair folded near the entrance; another, a child's drawing posted on the door, and in the third, there is a letter sticking out of the mailbox. Except for a piece of lacy white wrought-iron trim hanging from the gutter of the roof, the fourth looks empty. I peer inside the living room, level with the street. There is furniture around and everything is in place. The order has a forlorn stillness; even the toy fire engine sits in a corner unattended.

La Piedad filled me with notions of a poor Chicana who only in death is granted a touch of decorative splendor. Lila Burns has portrayed "these women" as well-meaning but ignorant. They know about food stamps but not about Medicaid.

Yet this neat little place looks like every garden apartment I have seen of the newly wed or recently separated woman. Open the door and the child can be seen; outside are others the child can play with and, best of all, the car can pull right up to the door with the groceries. The whole set-up is resolutely middle class.

Again, something doesn't click. "The poor Chicana" was a college student who lived in a comfortable home. Would this sort of woman give birth because "she has nothing else to do"?

Lila Burns has given me several names to contact. I skip over the doctors. I have had enough of male professionals. And females, too, with their bourgeois bias.

She mentioned a Sister Ann, a nurse-midwife who works in a family-planning clinic. The idea of speaking with a nun is intriguing. Husbands, lovers, children—these are not a part of a nun's life. Although she is married, the husband is manifest only in spirit. A nun nevertheless is not immune to a menstrual cramp. Nor can she ignore the pull of the womb contracting, pushing out its monthly flow, turning over, striving to expel an interior lining with every lunar cycle. To marry God is possible; to renounce her own flesh is not.

The Nuns

"I hope you're not shocked hearing this from a nun, but what bothers me most is the way the women just stay with the men. Why don't they divorce them is what I wonder."

Sister Ann is what you might call a "right-on" nun. So is Sister Tina, sitting at her feet with a two-drawer file cabinet as a backrest. Both sisters, who appear to be in their late thirties, are dressed in comfortable pants; their white turtleneck tops are covered by navy short-sleeved V-neck pullovers, updating their habits with a layered look. The flat shoes pulled up over the ankles by sturdy laces give the sisters the aura of movement women. Comfort is the guiding spirit in the family-planning offices of the public health building, where Sisters Ann and Tina work.

But for the missing loop around the top, the small cross hanging around the neck of each nun could be a feminist medallion sporting the symbol of woman so commonly employed to express sisterhood. But the picture of an enlarged fetus pinned to the wall of the cozy office reveals that the sisters are bonded less by feminist loyalties than by the sacrificial blood of the lamb. I am taken aback to see this kind of propaganda in a government-funded family-planning center.

The poster notwithstanding, I explain to the seated sisters that I have come to McAllen to find out about a woman who died after receiving an illegal abortion.

"You must tell her about the five young women with cancer of the uterus or breast," Sister Tina urges. "I think she will like that."

Sister Ann obliges by saying matter-of-factly, "Every one of the five was divorced within a year."

"You see, there is a sense here in McAllen in which sickness is viewed as a punishment for sex."

"It's much simpler than that. When the women get sick, the husbands leave. No need to bring in punishment or sin," Sister Ann says impatiently.

Sister Tina makes another offering. "I think this will interest you. There is a lot of superstition among the women. When there is a full moon or an eclipse, they wear a key pinned to the waist which they believe prevents damage to the baby, especially hare-lip."

Sister Ann gives Sister Tina a stern look, as if she does not approve of her attempts at appeasement. After all, she and I are on opposing sides of an issue fundamental to us both.

Sitting upright in her chair, Sister Ann talks about the early age at which the girls become sexually active. Her clinical manner includes frequent but incomplete references to numbers.

She says Hidalgo County has the third-highest VD rate but doesn't say where. It's clear, however, this is not Lila Burns's Hidalgo County where VD is "almost nonexistent." Sister Ann's litany resumes: life expectancy of a migrant worker is half that of a male professional, illegitimate babies are common, so is wife beating. It is all pretty grim.

As soon as Sister Ann mentions the high rate of teen-age pregnancy, Sister Tina returns to ritual, carrying on in a jovial manner about the celebration held for Mexican-American girls when they turn fifteen.

"It is very beautiful. Every member of the family, even distant ones, chip in and bring a present to the *quincineta*. Fifteen is the age when a girl officially turns into a woman, and what a splendid feast she has."

"Oh, Tina, that's why they make so many relatives godcousins when they are baptized. They know they can count on every last one to throw in a contribution."

It is becoming apparent that Sister Ann is a tough-minded thinker. There is something vaudevillian in the coupling of Sister Ann, the cynic, with Sister Tina, the sentimentalist.

I ask the pair what happens when the fifteen-year-old "woman" becomes pregnant.

"There is an expression, '*me esposo no quiero*,' which means 'my husband doesn't desire me.' "

"That is the literal translation, Tina. What they really mean is the man withdraws."

Sister Ann's tone of expertise invites speculation. Was she a wild one who used to run around with boys? There is something in her manner that makes me wonder whether she has converted her sexual curiosity into a service occupation, allowing her to openly explore what would otherwise remain taboo.

"Down here, to impregnate a woman is to be a man," Sister Ann says with a mixture of approval and contempt.

"Tell her, Ann, about the woman who became pregnant by the salamander."

Sister Ann, ignoring Tina, continues to offer figures on the high rate of rape, incest, and sex between juveniles and adults. "Recently, we had a case of a six-year-old who died after being raped by her mother's boyfriend. The man claimed he was getting back at the mother for rejecting him. He was not at all interested in the daughter sexually, he insisted."

"And now, Ann, the salamander," Sister Tina says, like a child who has patiently waited her turn.

In a perfunctory manner, Sister Ann relates the story of a fourteen-year-old-girl whose parents were convinced she became pregnant by a salamander. When Sister Ann says that actually it was a fifteen-year-old boy, Sister Tina guffaws as if she has just gotten the punch line of a joke.

Listening to the nuns is a little like reading the headlines of the *National Enquirer*. Although Sister Ann may be the tough-minded realist and Tina the fanciful one, both share an affinity for the sexually bizarre.

"What are you doing tonight?" Sister Tina inquires as the light from the outside fades. "If you have nothing planned, perhaps you would like to join us for dinner. It is a more comfortable setting at home, and we could show you some slides that I think would interest you."

I accept the sisters' invitation to dinner and get into my car. I've been instructed to follow them to the trailer park where they share a house with another nun.

Sister Tina is a mean driver. Not a bit of hesitation behind the wheel. I feel as if I'm following the Flying Nun as she flashes her directional before overtaking a truck loaded with green bananas.

We whiz past the City of Palms, where a billboard advertises Cassa Air Ambulances. It must be comforting to the "snowbirds" to know that, if moribund, they can be flown home.

As Sister Tina signals a righthand exit off the highway, another sign—this one for Loners on Wheels—looms ahead. A development of lonely amputees would fit right into the Texas mosaic. But Loners on Wheels does not refer to lonely people in wheelchairs; it is the term for elderly folk living alone in trailer camps.

I follow Sister Tina's car off the road, right up to the trailer camp, where we park beside a dwelling more substantial than anything on wheels. Inside the modest one-story brick house we are joined by Sister Jean, who asks what I would like to drink. I am not sure what is appropriate. Sensing my uncertainty, Sister Ann makes explicit the choices. I turn down the wine in favor of freshly squeezed orange juice.

The table has already been set by Sister Jean, who did not know about company. Without a word, she goes about lifting the settings and adding an extra place.

When we are all seated at the table, Sister Ann lowers her head to offer a benediction. After thanking the Lord for daily bread, she asks Him to help me obtain the information I am seeking. The sweetly pragmatic prayer embarrasses me; it doesn't seem right to call upon the Lord to collaborate in an abortion story. But I accept the blessing with the sincerity with which it is offered.

The sisters could almost be "role models" for women who live communally. Women with independent lives coming home every night to a relaxed meal set out with care but without excess fuss. Throughout the dinner, the sisters tease each other with a warm playfulness, arguing over who has the largest appetite, who is the most compulsive cleaner, and who has the hardest time getting up early in the morning. The harmony in their home could make it the envy of every counterculture commune, except that it's too aggressively innocent. For the moment, it could be a home in a TV commercial, except there are no men.

The nuns speak warmly of their families. Sister Tina comes from a large Italian family and Sister Ann is of Dutch descent. Sister Jean, the quiet one, is Eastern European. What is it like to be Jewish, they ask. I have never heard the question stated with such innocent curiosity.

After we clear the table, Sister Tina suggests we settle in for a slide show. Sister Jean promptly removes a Mexican fabric from the wall that now serves as a screen.

"I'm almost ready," Sister Tina cries out, as she fiddles with a slide carrousel.

"Whoopee, she's out of the closet," Ann exclaims.

"Okay, I confess I'm a closet photographer. No sin in that, is there?" Sister Tina asks, followed quickly by "Lights." Sister Jean jumps up and turns out the lights.

The first slide shows an old Mexican woman standing by a shingle hanging in front of a bungalow. Sister Tina focuses until a stork on the shingle becomes clear, explaining that the bird signifies the presence of a *partera*. I remember hearing the term before, when Doctor Garza referred to the lay Mexican midwives. Sister Tina says she prefers to think of them as "granny-midwives."

Sister Pat immediately produces figures: the average age of the *parteras* is eighty; 76 out of every 100 births in Brownsville are delivered by *parteras*, who are supposed to be licensed. Brownsville is the most popular border town for illegal aliens because the river is so narrow there, she says and then snaps "Next."

In the second slide, a *partera*, dressed in woolly knee socks, a loose dress, an apron, and an old sweater, is standing near a lumpy cot covered with newspapers and surrounded by two dogs and three birds in a cage. In one corner is a small altar and in another, a table with a pair of rusty-looking scissors and a scale, with a tray suspended by a hook on top. On the wall is a clock and a phone, next to which are printed, in large black letters, the names of the justice of the peace and the hospital, each with an adjacent telephone listing.

I flash back to the three cubicles in a bullfighting ring I once visited in Barcelona—a chapel, an operating room, and a morgue, all lined up behind the open arena.

As the slide show continues, the narration takes on the flavor of that of the salamander pregnancy. Luisa, the eighty-three-year-old *partera* with cataracts, has a positive VDRL. The thought of syphilis in an eighty-three-year-old woman seems to amuse Sister Tina as much as the cataracts alarm Sister Ann, who then carries on with an outrage not wholly without glee, telling us about Donna, an illiterate but fully sighted *partera* who cut an umbilical cord on Christmas Day with used dental floss, causing the baby to part not only from the mother but from the earth as well. Sister Tina then throws in the baby who died because of the rusty scissors.

Hearing their tales, I am perplexed by the popularity of the *parteras*. The sisters explain there are two main reasons. One is money: the *parteras* charge only one hundred dollars for a single birth and, in what I consider a charming display of literalness, two hundred for twins. Second, by signing birth certificates in the United States, the *parteras* can help grant dual citizenship to the babies of Mexican women—the real reason they are so popular, Sister Ann insists.

A nurse-midwife herself, Sister Ann is quite indignant about the *parteras*, vacillating between fury at their delivery techniques —"they actually massage the skin between the vagina and rectum with olive oil, which of course makes their hands more slippery" —and anger that they make a decent living—anywhere from twenty to twenty-five thousand dollars. "They will tell you they are supporting large families here and in Mexico. But how many times can you put your kids through college?"

Furthermore, if the woman doesn't have cash ahead of time, the *partera* will take anything she can get her hands on, even a cross. "I think they prefer watches to crosses," Sister Tina gently adds.

Skipping over the issue of payment, I ask if there's a way to teach them to boil a pair of scissors.

"We are trying to institute classes. But it is hard. The women are old and used to their own ways. They are afraid of dealing with any health authorities. Many are superstitious and believe that if a baby dies, it was meant to be."

I do not know how to respond to Sister Tina's remark. It seems to me she is not without her own sense of inevitability.

I think back to the clean antiseptic office of Dr. Chester. Even if a poor Mexican woman had the money for a doctor, how intimidating it must be for her to go there and perhaps to a hospital ward; how much more reassuring to give birth in the home of a grandmotherly *partera*, surrounded by religious mementos and herbal teas, letting God, in conjunction with nature, decide the destiny of the mother and child. I think of the long lists of what a woman on welfare must bring to Dr. Garza if she doesn't have her welfare card. The "grannys" do not operate in conditions too different from those on the communes, except that the young women delivering babies in the company of beards, dogs, roosters, and toddlers, do know how to sterilize scissors.

When Sister Tina finishes with the slides, I offer to help wash the dishes. Sister Ann explains that there is a system. "We have it so well worked out, we don't even think about it," she adds.

Sister Tina starts to give me instructions for getting back in the dark, then quite spontaneously she decides to lead the way. There is a drizzle and it is hard to see, she says when I protest.

I keep my eye on Sister Tina as she speeds along ahead of me. The license plate is from the Northwest, courtesy of a religious order. So is her home. The sisters are comfortably supported by the Church. For all their disdain of worldly goods, they have total economic security. Yet they condemn the "grannys" for their shiny American cars. The only way not to be a sinner is to be poor. With poverty comes compassion.

Of all the people I have met so far, the nuns come the closest to being comrades. And yet, the one area that dominates the lives of the women they see—men—is the one they never deal with themselves. For them, it is simple. Get rid of the men, divorce them, leave them, desert them.

In a perversely logical extension of Dr. Chester's dictum, the sisters are women who have learned how to say no.

Once back in my room, I take inventory. The *parteras* are an interesting story. Although I do not think they are real villains (the doctors who charge too much money and the county health officials who license *parteras* without training them come far closer) it does seem shocking that they can function legally in such unsanitary conditions.

Equally shocking, there is no place where a college student can comfortably find out the various means of birth control. "We don't actively recruit the young," Lila Burns said. The nuns who run the family-planning clinics display blown-up fetuses. And the few doctors who face the question push the pill.

I think someone should investigate the *parteras*. Had I the time, I would. Lacking it, I decide to call Chuck Duncan, a reporter for the ABC affiliate in Dallas, who did a gutsy story on the Mexican pharmacy where Rosie had her fatal abortion, which reminds me that, though I had learned about *parteras*, I did not learn anything about Rosie.

FOUR **DIANE**

The sign in front of Don Pepe's stand advertises *tacos,* breakfast *nachos,* and *enchiladas;* the slithery white stream against a red background assures the potential customer of a Coke. I make a left turn and suddenly there it is—Pan American University. Maybe it's my northern eye, accustomed to density, that finds buildings in the middle of nowhere a shock.

The young men and women walking hurriedly along the treeless concrete paths connecting the low beige stucco structures could be veterans and their wives returning to a postwar garden development erected in cheap imitation of Southwest architecture. But instead of bags of groceries, they carry books. Among the faculty is the sociology professor whose name Lila Burns has given me.

Juan Chavira, short, slender, with gentle tired eyes and a thick mustache, is wearing a woolly sweater and denims. He is not disturbed that I am late. Once I am seated in the office of the sociologist, I ask who is the militant Chicano looking down from the poster hanging on the wall. He laughs gently. "That word, *Chicano.* It isn't used much down here, although it is popular up North with intellectuals."

After a few more pleasantries are exchanged, I bring up Rosaura Jimenez. He is not familiar with the name. "The woman who died from an illegal abortion." Juan thinks for a while. Yes, he vaguely recalls the incident; however, it did not make much of an impression.

"But she was a student here. How about the school paper? Did it take note? Did they run an article about it?"

Juan puts his hand under his chin and closes his eyes. "I can't recall an article, but I will check for you. I'm pretty sure I would remember if there was one. But who knows. Let me see," Juan says, walking to a file cabinet. I give him the date of her death as he flips through back issues of the school paper. "Nothing about the abortion death from what I can see."

I tell Juan I don't have much time left; I am leaving tomorrow. "I wanted to find someone who really knew her. The only person I met who did was her personal physician, and he was not interested in talking."

I feel certain the registrar would know who her teachers were, but I am not so certain that the registrar would disclose that information to a stranger.

Juan offers to call, sparing me the awkwardness of a request. "I am flattered to help you investigate her death," he says, looking through a university directory for the extension of the registrar.

"What was her name?" Juan asks, as he picks up the telephone.

"Rosaura. Rosaura Jimenez," I say slowly.

"Ji-*men*-ez. The accent is on the second syllable," Juan says as he starts to dial. "Rosaura Jimenez," he repeats to himself. "No, the name definitely is not familiar," he says out loud.

"Her personal doctor called her Rosie," I toss in.

"Rosie? Wait a minute. I just thought of something." Juan slams down the receiver. "My god, I wonder if it could be the same woman. I'll be right back," he says, rushing out of the room.

Juan returns with a number scribbled on a piece of paper. "In just a minute we will know if it's the same," he says with excitement. "I had a research assistant last summer. Just this last week she dropped by to chat. I asked her how things were going. 'Well, not so good,' she says. 'My best friend died.' When I asked her if it was anyone I knew, all she said was, 'Her name was Rosie.' In just a minute we will know if it's the same person," he says.

Probably not, I say to myself, as I watch Juan waiting for an answer. She's not even home, I conclude. But then I hear Juan talking.

"We are in luck," Juan says to me as he puts down the receiver. "The woman you call Rosaura was the same person Diane told me about. The one who died. Rosie. That's her name."

I had thought the time spent with Homer a waste. Yet without it, I never would have known about the name Rosie.

"Do you think she'll speak with me?"

"Why don't you ask her yourself? Here, use the phone," Juan says, motioning me over to his desk.

I introduce myself and very simply ask the stranger on the phone if it is possible to meet with her to talk about Rosie.

"Yes, but I have only one hour between classes tomorrow," she says apologetically. Her voice is weak. Perhaps she isn't ready to talk; perhaps it's still too raw. I am not certain whether to press her.

"If you don't mind coming to my house, we could meet this afternoon," she adds, surprising me.

I wonder if she feels obliged to speak to me because of Juan.

The address she gives me sounds familiar. Hibiscus Street. I realize it is the same garden-apartment complex as Rosie's. Diane lives next door.

The sparse, cramped apartment reminds me of student housing —cheap stereo, handmade bookshelves, worn furniture, a pole lamp. Diane, taller and more composed than I expected from her mournful telephone voice, moves gracefully toward her chair and offers me a seat. She has long black hair that turns upward slightly at its ends. Her fair skin makes her look more Italian—northern Italian—than Mexican. Her tight, slender neck, narrow calves, long thin arms with the muscles clearly defined, sensuous rather than athletic, give her the appearance of an arty New England debutante—"a Sarah Lawrence or Bennington girl." Except for her sharply plucked eyebrows.

There is an appealing contrast between the composed, almost taut body and her tentative manner. It is hard to hear her—her voice is barely above a whisper—but I sense she wants to talk. Badly. First about herself.

"My parents made me believe I could never do anything right. I never liked going to pick tomatoes at ten cents a pound. They made me feel like there was something wrong, something peculiar with me, for resenting the work. But I thought why should I pick tomatoes for ten cents a pound for someone else to sell them for thirty-nine cents a pound—God, I don't want to do this for the rest of my life. My father would beat me up when I wouldn't go into the fields.

"Then I got asthma which, I guess, was the only way I had of protesting. The doctor told my family it's in my head. But I could see that it took so much work for them to earn any money and then it would be spent in one day just to keep us fed. This is not what I want. I see other people. They don't have to do this.

"As long as I can remember, I never liked being poor. All applications always said, 'What do your parents do?' I decided that when I had a child, he wasn't going to write in 'migrant worker.'

"At first, I wanted to be beautiful, a model. But can you see a model picking tomatoes? I wanted to go to school. They were always taking us out of school when we were in the fields.

"But that's where I met my husband. When we got married, I had more money, but I still had to stay home and have kids. I wasn't so good at that either. I have Rh-negative blood so I messed that one up, according to him.

"I was with him officially for four years, but actually for nine months. I didn't love him—he was too conceited. He went to Vietnam after Anthony was born. Had I stayed married, I'd have five kids by now, I'm sure. But I got divorced in July 1973, and started secretarial school in September. That's where I met Rosie.

"She took me out to a restaurant and said we have to stand on our own two feet. Rosie changed my life. She was the one who talked me into going to college. We both had little children and I wasn't so sure. But Rosie said, 'We have to; we have to become independent.'

"Her family didn't talk to her for a long time when she had the child. I used to lend her money. She was real poor. But she was the one who would cheer me up. She'd say, 'We Leos are queens. We can't settle for this stuff.'

"She was always pretending to be rich. She went out with a lot of guys because she wanted someone to care for her. She would go out with a guy once, and if he treated her well—you know, took her to a nice restaurant, didn't mind her kid being around—she would say, 'He's in love with me,' and then she would get her hopes up high. And it was like she was two different people, because another part of her believed so much that the only way she could change her life was to get her degree and be independent. If it weren't for her, I wouldn't be in school now. Neither would Margie; she lives here too and also has a young boy.

"You see, Rosie had this knowledge. It was like a vision. She had to get away. When she was fifteen, her mother left her with beans to cook and the beans burned. The mother came home and hit her hard. Rosie went to the police and tried to turn herself in. She didn't want to go back home. But the sad thing is I don't think she ever got over the rejection. She was still trying to get her parents to accept her. Or some substitute. And because she knew what it was like not to be loved, she tried desperately to be a good mother to Jenny, her daughter. She wanted to be somebody real bad. I think she was grasping real hard for life.

"We didn't want to work in the fields, Rosie and me. We didn't even want to be secretaries. I said to my mother, 'What about the future of my child?' when she would try to talk me out of any fancy dreams—or what she considered fancy dreams. See, here's where Rosie helped me. The biggest thing was going to school. That's what she said we had to concentrate on.

"My father is a drunk, a no-good bum, and I was the oldest of seven daughters. When I told my mother about wanting to go to college, she said, 'It's a waste of money. You shouldn't be doing that. Find a husband.' But my first husband beat me up so bad that I knew that was no solution. I was determined to survive. And even though my mother didn't approve, she still didn't throw me out.

"If I didn't have my little boy, I wouldn't have lasted this long. It's a funny thing. It's impossible with him around, but he keeps

me going. He's like my reason to stay as determined. I can't stop.
I can't give up. Even when I want to for myself, I have him to
remember.

"Rosie was the same way with Jenny. Even more so.

"I was pretty low just after I had my own baby and was trying to make ends meet. When we started school, that's when
everything changed. It was a different world. Like our ex-boss
from secretarial school used to call us college coeds. Rosie
would say, 'It's too bad we can't live in dorms like real college
students.'

"I could have gone the same route as Rosie did, but I had a
mother who supported me even though she didn't understand
me. She would be scared if I told her I'm studying to be a lawyer.
But she would understand if I had a job packing vegetables in a
warehouse. The other doesn't make any sense to her. It doesn't
seem real.

"But Rosie kept on encouraging me to keep with it.

"She was like someone I wanted to be. She was happy. I was
pessimistic. Nothing upset her, or *seemed* to. She could strike up
a conversation with anyone. She is me in the future, I thought
—I've already gone through what she has. We live a couple of
lives.

"Rosie and I were in secretarial school until September 1974.
They kept trying to kick us out. We were too smart. 'Well, you're
ready to get a job,' they'd say. And we kept sticking around the
school. It was a government-sponsored program to train women
to be secretaries, so we didn't have to pay. But we didn't want
to be secretaries. We wanted to stay in school. It was like a way
of erasing the past, getting an education.

"We met this fantastic lady, Esther. She was secretary of the
secretarial school. That sounds like a joke, doesn't it? She was
happily married, but she told us, 'Not everyone is lucky. Why
don't you plan to do something important with your lives?'

"Finally, Rosie and I got the courage to enroll in college. We
both got scholarships and started at Pan Am. At first I felt out
of place. I thought people in college could tell I was dumber than
they. But Rosie would say, 'Oh, come on.' She acted like she had

been there all her life. She would constantly tell me to loosen up. 'Let's go out night-clubbing.' I was excited about it but scared. Sitting there with a bunch of kids and all they think about is getting drunk and having fun, and all I'm thinking about is how I'm going to get the money to eat. And she was having fun, going out with high-class guys. She would introduce me to them, and they would say, 'Nice piece,' like a piece of furniture. After a while I stopped going. It was too uncomfortable.

"Any attention Rosie got, she enjoyed. This guy followed her down the hall. She would tell me, 'He must really like me.' He might have just been going the same way, but she couldn't believe it. That's how lonely she really was. But she never felt herself getting lonely. I was seeing a psychiatrist, I was so depressed. She would infect you with her laughter. 'Oh, that's the psychologist in you,' she would say if ever I pointed out another side to her gaiety.

"My therapist didn't really understand either. He used to tell me, 'You should be a secretary, you're so good looking.'

"Rosie went out with young guys always. She felt she was too old, that she missed something along the way, and now she was trying to make up for it. Except for the doctor she was friendly with. She used to confide in him. He was older and married. But he also tried to act like a kid, like some hippie, you know, not a doctor. He could afford to take her to nice places which she liked. To her it was a sign of love. And he didn't charge her for visits, she said.

"Seeing Rosie look so happy, even though I knew there was another side, made me feel peculiar. I tried to commit suicide. Not because I wanted to die but because I was feeling so alone.

"Rosie had a lot of friends. She needed people around her— girlfriends, boyfriends, all colors. She went out with a lot of guys. It wasn't sex so much. She would say, 'He brought me a rose. He took me to a restaurant.' It was as if everything she knew in her head she would forget when a guy showed her any attention or was even nice to her. She was one of those laughing-on-the-outside, crying-on-the-inside people. She loved having her picture taken. She was really peppy looking and she was active in the

Future Teachers Club. She wanted to teach disturbed children. And I took up psychology because of my little boy. Margie and I have hyperactive kids, like Rosie did.

"Rosie liked all kinds of people. I am much shyer, I guess. My mother told me, don't let a boy touch you hard. You'll get pregnant. So I got married, just to get out of the house. And I went from one prison to another, except this one was worse because I had a baby. That's why I never understood why Rosie wanted to get married so bad.

"I mean I did understand it on one level. Her family had always made her feel so ashamed about having a baby when she wasn't married. When she was pregnant and the whole family was going out one time, Rosie got dressed up, and as they were leaving, her father said, 'What are you doing; you can't go out. No one is going to see I have a whore for a daughter.'

"My parents weren't like that, but I still felt so alone.

"Then I met a guy on Christmas Eve. The guy I'm living with now. He is a typical Mexican-American guy, *machismo* and all, but I know he loves me. When I'm sick or whatever, he brings me breakfast in bed. But he just can't stand the idea that I want to be a lawyer. Sometimes he asks, 'And what am I going to be, your assistant?' He's very sensitive about my education because he never graduated from high school. He shows me off and tells everyone I'm going to be a lawyer, but underneath he resents it when he's not bragging.

"And things looked good for Rosie, too. She had a new boyfriend, Jesse. He was Mexican-American and he had a little girl too. Both of the children would play together. It was the first serious steady boyfriend Rosie had. He owned some land which he was going to sell when she graduated, and they were going to get married and move out of McAllen. Away. But then Jesse got into trouble and landed in jail.

"He was twenty-eight and on probation for drugs or something. They had revoked his probation and sent him to prison after she was sort of living with him for one year. They took him away one month before the abortion.

"Before Jesse, Rosie never had anyone to share her aspirations with. Jesse wanted Rosie to have a child. His, of course. And then she got pregnant by somebody else.

"Rosie was scared. She wanted someone who could take care of her, and Jesse was in jail. She was always taking care of others. She was super-responsible with her little girl.

"At least my boyfriend takes care of Anthony when I have to study for an exam, or my mother will take him for a day or two. But Rosie had no backup like that. She was all alone, especially after Jesse went to jail.

"She was reluctant at first to admit how much she cared about him, because the more she cared, the more vulnerable it made her feel—and she was very vulnerable to start with.

"After he left, she started going out with guys left and right. There was this one guy she was seeing who owns this head shop. Just a little rich boy, and, of course, she fell for that, even though it wasn't anything serious.

"I think she really did love Jesse. She went to see him in jail up in Houston two weeks before she died. He was going to file for divorce from his first wife so they could get married. Rosie always wanted to get married. That was her dream. She started going to church, not the Catholic church but to a pastor in the Baptist church. I think she was covering up a depression and was comforted by the idea of being born again. She was very anxious.

"Her sister was going to make a white wedding dress for her. That is what they buried her in, I think. I didn't go to the funeral, but they say she looked real bad even though they tried to fix her up.

"Her relatives wanted to blame me for what happened. I wanted to tell this lady, her mother, 'Look, if you had loved her a little more . . .' but I couldn't talk to her. It was like trying to get through to a stone wall. Such hypocrites, I thought. They didn't show their love when she was alive and needed it, and now all this crying and carrying on. They all came down from Houston to McAllen and were standing in the street screaming at one another. The mother went out hunting for her husband every night. Meanwhile, Rosie was in the hospital dying.

"Once I said to Rosie, before she got sick, 'Rosie, how can you stand it?' 'She's my mother,' is all she said. She really did not want to face that she was rejected. Her mother was pretty shot, I guess. She had twelve children and they were real poor. Her father used to have a hamburger stand right on the highway. All the kids were in and out of trouble. I know it wasn't easy for her mother, but still. . . .

"The whole thing has taught me how important it is not to reject your children. That's why I'm going to do everything I can to see that I'm a good mother to Anthony, even though he drives me crazy."

Diane sighs, pauses. She has been talking—intensely, quietly— for almost an hour.

"I think the pregnancy was the last straw for Rosie. For so long she had pretended that she was happy. The pregnancy tipped everything. She could no longer pretend. She already had one child. She really loved Jenny, but it was hard. She was on welfare for eighty-six dollars a month, taking care of Jenny all by herself and going to college and working part time. I know Rosie would not have had the illegal abortion if she had money. And I guess, with Jesse in jail, the one person who really did love her at last . . . it's like suddenly she let her defenses down and just gave up."

Abruptly Diane stops. She becomes quiet, as if she is listening for something.

As I stare at her tailored shirt, partially opened, it is almost impossible to think that, less than ten years ago, she was picking tomatoes for ten cents a pound. Her stare is both despairing and pensive.

It is as if we've been under a spell, the lives of two women alternating so rapidly they seem to fuse. Except one lives, the other doesn't: "I could have gone the same route as Rosie did . . ."

Both tried to juggle two dreams: the desire to be protected, taken care of ("We Leos are queens") and the need to be autonomous ("We have to stand on our own two feet"). But neither seemed to have the single-mindedness it takes to survive on one's own. Neither seemed ruthless or determined enough. It takes a

tougher attitude and a greater sense of self to resolve the conflicting desires.

Diane fingers a delicate gold chain around her neck. Her jew-
eled watch fits the part that wants to be a model. There is a
sadness that Diane, already a bit weary and defeated, seems aware
of but doesn't articulate: that Rosie, who changed her life, who
"was like someone I wanted to be," is dead. And Diane, who tried
to kill herself "because I was so alone," is alive.

It is as if she lived, but just barely.

And why did it have to be Rosie who died? Because the mother
rejected her? Or because the government cut off Medicaid? For
Diane, who "took up psychology," it's the mother who's to blame.
Yet she says, "Rosie would not have had the illegal abortion if she
had money."

I still don't know.

"Stop it, Anthony," Diane screams as someone kicks open the
door. It is a shock to hear her yell; during the nonstop recitation,
she showed little emotion.

The conversation reverts to a normal dialogue. We spend some
time discussing her courses. Her favorite is women's studies. She
goes to find the reading list. "Only women," she says. I look over
the names: Willa Cather, Margaret Atwood, Carson McCullers,
an anthology of women poets, *Rising Tides.* "When you came I
was reading *The Bell Jar.* Maybe that is why I felt like opening
up. I was thinking of Rosie while I was reading that book, and
of my own life too. I just realized I haven't asked you anything
about yourself. I'm sorry, I was so involved with our lives."

We hug awkwardly and I talk about my own life, the abortion
I had before it was legal. Diane promises to send me a list of the
feminist books she cannot get in McAllen. I will send them along
with pamphlets on contraception. We spend a moment trying to
figure out how to send a diaphragm in the mail.

"That will be great. Most of my friends have never even seen
one. All the doctors do is write a prescription for pills."

I pick up a copy of Dr. Spock in Spanish. Diane looks embarrassed. "You can see I was just starting out. I wasn't even up to
English in those days."

"Do you know his wife helped him to write that book?"

"I always wondered how a man could know so much about kids. He's not the one who stays home with them all day.

"There's this book they sell in the book store at school called *Club and Sword*. It's supposed to be for Mexican-American women. It says they like to be beaten by their husbands because it's a sign of love. The women are all mad about that.

"I collect books. Anything I can get," she says. "I just read Sue Kaufman's *Diary of a Mad Housewife*."

I tell Diane that Kaufman's second book was called *Falling Bodies* and that the author jumped out of her window one summer day.

"To me she seemed to have everything you would ever want. But even when a woman seems so different, I try to understand because I know that to others my life and Rosie's looks real easy. Like we have everything—cars, clothes, we go out. That's all they see. But," she says, "I am a feminist and . . ." Hesitating, she adds, "So was Rosie. In her way."

During May of 1977, the world's largest biological warfare program was launched. Every day pilots took off from Mission, Texas. The target—the screwworm fly. Four hundred million males, each sterilized by an atomic weapon—a cesium-137 isotope—were dropped from C-45's. It was thought that the sterile male flies would breed with fertile females and produce zero population.

Four miles from the Screwworm Eradication Center in Mission is the McAllen Airport. A few yards from the runway is La Piedad, park of buried bones and mesquite trees; the soil of the cemetery absorbs the fallout of fertility gone amok.

There are no seat reservations on Texas International's flight out of McAllen. As soon as passengers are allowed to board, I take a window seat on the right-hand side. Take-off involves a minimum of fuss. There are the customary remarks: Oxygen masks are located above the seats in the event that . . . Please observe the no smoking sign until . . .

And then I see Rosie right by the runway, her graveside belly bloated with ribbons. The Styrofoam cross has been knocked down and thrown over her grave. A protective gesture.

The plane is gaining altitude. I take one last look at her still-new covering before the coronas are replaced by giant cotton puffs as McAllen disappears beneath the clouds.

PART 2

THE GOVERNMENT ENTERS THE INVESTIGATION (AGAIN)

FIVE **RETURN TO MCALLEN**

"There's new information about Rosie. I think it's important. I'll try to call you again."

I recognized the soft voice on the answering machine as Diane's and phoned her back right away.

The new information stunned me. Rosie hadn't had the abortion in Mexico. She'd had it in McAllen. I had no chance to respond. In her quiet, quick style, Diane explained that a friend of Rosie's named Evangelina had called Pauline, the sister of Rosie's fiancé; Evangelina had told Pauline that she was the only one who knew what had really happened. After hearing all the lies on television, Evangelina felt she could no longer remain silent —even though her psychiatrist had warned she might have another nervous breakdown if she talked about Rosie.

She confessed that she had taken Rosie to Maria Pineda, a McAllen *partera*. She had stayed that Sunday night while Maria Pineda performed the abortion in her home. The following evening Rosie was in intensive care, and Evangelina, shortly afterward, was hospitalized for a nervous breakdown.

Diane didn't know Evangelina's number but suggested that I get it from Rosie's intended sister-in-law, Pauline. I called Pauline who, in a firm tone, repeated the story just as Diane had told it. She went on to add the most critical information. Rosie had had an abortion in January or February of 1977, paid for by Medicaid. She had been referred to a private medical group in Harlingen by McAllen Planned Parenthood. It was now clear that Rosie had had her abortion with Maria Pineda because she could not afford a doctor. The idea that she was motivated by shame was incorrect. This, I felt, could be the turning point of the investigation.

If what the women said could be verified, every report so far —by the CDC, Califano, Carter, Chester, Homer Rivas, Lila Burns, "Good Morning America," *Ob.Gyn. News, The New York Times,* the *Washington Post,* the *Boston Globe,* and the *Los Angeles Times*—was wrong.

Although the government had never come up with a witness or any documentary evidence, it had never questioned that Rosie went to Mexico for her fatal abortion; only her motivation had been in dispute.

Yet the CDC doctors had not used tentative language when they wrote up their findings for the official report published by the United States Department of Health, Education and Welfare, November 4, 1977:

> . . . A 27-year-old woman was hospitalized September 26th, 1977, with symptoms of fever, knee pain, and lower abdominal pain. . . . On September 1st and September 9th she had consulted her physician about sternal pain. On the second visit, when she indicated to her physician that she might be pregnant, he informed her that Medicaid no longer paid for abortions. She subsequently obtained an induced abortion in Mexico. . . .

When the CDC published this account of Rosie's death, Dr. Julian Gold was the chief government investigator on the scene. He was the one who had started the original round of publicity, and although only a junior epidemiology officer, he had been held responsible for the government's account, by *Ob.Gyn. News,* a semi-monthly medical newspaper published by Fairchild for obstetricians and gynecologists.

In a copyrighted story in the December 1, 1977, issue of *Ob. Gyn. News,* Dr. Gold was accused of covering up that the dead woman "had gone to Mexico two years ago" for an illegal abortion, even though Medicaid was available at the time.

The allegations against Dr. Gold printed by *Ob.Gyn. News*

(which has a more conservative readership than does the *MMWR*, the CDC weekly where Dr. Gold's report first appeared) were based on interviews with Homer Rivas and Lila Burns; both confirmed they would have arranged a free or low-cost legal abortion if only "the dead woman" had sought their help before going to Mexico. Both expressed dismay that she hadn't when they were interviewed by telephone.

Rivas further told the reporters that, as Rosie's personal physician, he was in a position to know that, even when Medicaid funds were available for abortion in 1975, she chose not to use them and had gone instead to Mexico where she had her first of three abortions—the one Dr. Gold was accused of covering up. With Lila Burns echoing him, Rivas pointed out that it is not uncommon for Mexican-American women to cross the border because of feelings of shame, ending on a note of inevitability common to Greek choruses. "We had this problem long before Medicaid abortions and we'll have it long afterwards."

Although the *Ob.Gyn.* article raised serious doubts about Dr. Gold's credibility, he stood behind his original story, stating that his conclusions were based on extensive on-site interviews; besides, there was no hard data to back up the claims of Rivas and Burns that "the dead woman" had gone across the border even when there was Medicaid money available for an abortion.

That data had now been provided by Pauline. If Lila Burns had checked her referral files at Planned Parenthood, she, too, could have provided it. Why hadn't the CDC unearthed this fact in its first investigation?

Years ago, when I was studying philosophy, questions of *what* the world is made of interested me less than *how we know* what the world is made of. By what process do we come to think of something as true? Such concerns are often abstract. With Rosie, epistemology had come alive.

According to the logical positivists I had studied, the only statements with meaning are those that can be verified. All statements of faith or feeling are without logical sense; are, in fact, non-sense. While maintaining a guarded respect for the strict sense of meaning supplied by the positivists, I have never accepted it as the *only* definition of meaning. Feelings, intuitions, while more elusive, have always seemed to strengthen what I could know by the verifiable, objective methods we've come to call "science."

My intuitions told me that what Diane and Pauline had said was the truth. But I knew it was imperative to document my feelings with facts. Although guilty itself of equating feelings with facts, the government would never accept the hearsay of women, especially poor, nonwhite women.

What the women said contradicted what the white middle-class professionals, with whom the CDC doctors identified, said. What's more, the official government report had been accepted, without question, by all the media, including those that pride themselves on their objectivity.

By now I had a first-hand knowledge of CDC "methodology." In four months of interviews it never once occurred to CDC officers to talk to women who knew Rosie. Their official reports were based entirely on interviews with their own peers.

Although the government's behavior was sexist and racist, I do not believe it was consciously so. I phoned CDC to tell them the new information. I had already decided to return to McAllen when I was invited to accompany the government team. I thought back to my first Texas trip, when the CDC officials would not even release the name of the woman whose death I was investigating. "Classified information," they had said. Things had obviously reversed themselves. Since I had learned the identity of the abortionist and the fact of a prior Medicaid abortion, the investigators assumed a more humble approach: perhaps we could work together. I agreed to fly to McAllen and "work together." We would interview Maria Pineda, the abortionist, and Evangelina, the witness; we would also try to document Rosie's previous abortion history.

The second investigation of Rosaura Jimenez's death began on February 12, 1978, four months after her death on October 3,

1977, three months after the first government report of November 4, and ten days after I had met Diane.

Now I was to continue my work with the EIS officers of the ASB, FPED, CDC, HEW. Not only did I have misgivings about working with government officials, I also don't trust the cryptic. Unpronounceable names, like the organizations they stand for, are part of a secret code, moving toward mystification at the same velocity they move away from comprehensibility. Who knows for sure what they stand for?

Take CDC. A *C* could stand for congressional, constitutional, company, committee, even Columbia. But the *C* in this instance stands for Center, the *D* for Disease, and the second *C* cagily repeated only in letter, for Control. CDC. Center for Disease Control. Even with the full name known, few have any idea of what, if anything, the CDC is supposed to *do*.

What's more, this branch of the federal government, located not in Washington, but down in Atlanta, publishes the *MMWR* every week. Even a lover of acronyms might stumble over *MMWR: The Mortality and Morbidity Weekly Report.* Keep it in mind; it chronicles the course of diseases being looked into by doctors turned detectives, hot on the trail of mysterious microbes that manage to slip across borders without passports, moving from country to country, from body to body, from cell to cell, spreading fear and contagion.

Of course, abortion is not a disease. Yet the CDC has an active abortion-surveillance program, a program that was established only after much in-fighting and bureaucratic maneuvering. In 1969, three staff members in the Family Planning Evaluation Division, John Asher, M.D., Judith Bourne Rooks, R.N., and Carl Tyler, M.D. (now FPED director), recognized that illegal abortions were a major public health hazard to women. Mortality and morbidity resulting from illegal abortion were alarmingly high. This was particularly true for poor women. The three CDC officials felt that a major obligation of the CDC was to evaluate such public health problems, even ones so highly controversial.

They developed and fought for a rationale for CDC involvement in this area: unwanted pregnancy was termed a disease that, like VD, was sexually transmitted. Again and again, the three came close to losing their jobs for pursuing what we now see as the pioneering but mild study of illegal-abortion complications. Their commitment to that study helped the Supreme Court to understand the importance of affirming a woman's constitutional right to safe, legal abortion. But ultimately the CDC suffered from the problem of all bureaucracy—when you have won a difficult battle, you retrench, you take fewer risks. Eventually, you may forget that you were originally concerned with a real problem—women dying from illegal abortions—and come to distort your rationale. Now the CDC had regressed to viewing abortion as the disease, instead of unwanted pregnancy.

SIX THE CDC TEAM

The group of young doctors, sent to Texas by the CDC after my call, were different from those I had talked to in McAllen. Sons of the sixties, they were equally suspicious of organizations whose work remains furtive. Having chosen to revive the ancient tradition of public health service, they do not deal with private patients and modes of payment. Instead of the paraphernalia of commerce, they carry knapsacks filled with good intentions. They know that the poor receive worse treatment than the rich. They know that is wrong. To them, abortion is a "social disease."

"It's all class," Mark Nelson says when we meet at La Posada. "It would be a mistake to place the blame on men." At first, I am suspicious; men who worry about being blamed often have problems with feminists. But since Mark has none of the arrogance of most doctors, male or female, I withhold judgment. He is a male feminist, but thank God he doesn't proclaim himself one.

Assigned to Texas by the CDC, he is a public health officer who has come down to McAllen from Austin. He tells me that throughout the sixties politics was his passion. Then he went into analysis. Rosie is important to Mark. Her story touches everything of current interest to him—sexual roles, control over one's body, the mystique of medicine. But mainly, he concludes, it is a case of social injustice.

He seems attracted to suffering, which worries me. His identification is with women—their emotionality, their ability to feel. He doesn't trust the local doctors; he thinks Dan Chester is obtuse. He questions his bosses, his job, his life. He is a quester, not yet locked into the convent of careerism. Mark, at thirty, still dreams of changing the world, but first he would like to understand it. He is willing, even anxious, to learn from women.

His colleague, Julian Gold, is also hip to the times. Unlike Mark, who thinks in terms of sublimation, Julian is not impressed by the Freudian hierarchy. Who says genital functioning is higher than oral? Who says sex must end in orgasm inside the vagina? What about sex for warmth and affection? Wives for friendship and passion? And for aggression, what about work?

Julian's head of dark curls, his bearded face with deep-set blue eyes and droopy lids, lends a soft sensuality to his appearance. A fierce competitiveness is belied by his transparent Indian shirt, delicate silver chains, and tight pants that flare at the cuffs. Son of an Australian millionaire, Julian Gold is married to a strong, independent woman who works in theater. We met when I was a guest at their elegant commune in Atlanta. He knows exactly what he wants to be—another Schweitzer—and he knows that such a lofty ambition is enhanced by softening touches.

Dr. Ward Cates, five years older than his two colleagues, is the last of the CDC trio. Not quite comfortable with the offbeat, he overlooks it as Julian openly, defiantly cultivates it and Mark observes it from a slight distance. The highest in rank, Ward is the most conventional—suggesting the link Mark suspects and Julian ignores between conformity and advancement within a hierarchy.

Ward has the sunny look and gentlemanly manner one associates with earnest preppies. He is married, has two children, loves his work and his wife, doesn't drink or turn on, and doesn't judge those who do. For, above all, Ward loves tolerance, especially in others.

Combing through hospital charts, tracking down strange organisms pleases Ward. But not Julian, who joined the Public Health Service in search of adventure. It matters little that as a foreigner he cannot be ranked. He is willing to forego all appellations and be labeled "visiting scientist" instead of "captain" or "lieutenant," as long as he is not confined to working with figures.

Mark, too, is interested in the human drama. But he feels inhibited about expressing his interest openly, although not as inhibited as Ward. For who, it could be argued, would not wish to get a look at a person involved in a death he had been investigating for months. Although morally respectable, it is emotionally unconvincing to prefer to sit in the record room of a hospital monitoring dates of admission and dates of release (whether to the morgue or home).

This then was the government team—borderline hip, borderline square, and flamboyant adventurer.

SEVEN **MARIA PINEDA**

Monday, the morning after our arrival, we meet in the La Posada coffee shop to discuss how to contact Maria Pineda. Julian suggests we visit her together. I point out that she will become suspicious if men are involved. I am already concerned about how she will react to the face of an Anglo woman.

Julian will not pretend he prefers to read about Maria Pineda than to see her. He is raring to go. I have the feeling it is the first time his gender has been an obstruction. Until now, being a man has been an asset; it has eased his entry into doctors' offices and the oval rooms of office holders. Dan Chester enjoys playing a game of tennis with his colleague, after talking over "the case." Reporters from *Ob.Gyn. News* try hard to reach Dr. Julian Gold on the telephone for a comment.

Acutely aware of Julian's disappointment at being left out, I make an effort to include him as much as the situation allows. We pile into a car—Julian's, not mine—to case out Maria Pineda's neighborhood together, leaving the "winter Texans" behind at La Posada.

With Julian up front and Mark in the back, we drive past the blinking-yellow at the railroad crossing and turn onto the business highway parallel to the tracks, past the once strange warehouses, now grown familiar. At the end of the row of warehouses is the turn for Reynosa. Instead of taking it, we make a right and enter a new neighborhood—one entirely Mexican, although it is only a few blocks from La Posada.

Instead of names like Pecan, Ivy, Magnolia, Hibiscus, the

streets have numbers. Rosie's move from North Nineteenth to Hibiscus—away from the literal toward the abstract, where a number becomes a name and a name becomes a symbol—mirrors the evolution of intelligence and urban sprawl.

When there is more money, it is not essential to accumulate streets numerically with the railroad track as the starting point. Even Hibiscus is not the end of aspiration. With really big bucks, you can live at a place where the home is so large it *is* the address. At King Ranch you don't need a number or even a street.

I notice that the neighborhood supermarket has an oblong-shaped marquee with the letters R-I-V-A-S running down the length. It is part of the chain owned by Homer's family. Larger than a neighborhood store, it does not have the vast spread of the Family Mall Shopping Center, although it *is* the family shopping center, no matter what the developers say. What's more, just as Homer boasted, the supermarket does take food stamps for beer and cigarettes, although it is against the law to do so.

Next to the Rivas supermarket are houses similar to those on the *colonias*—unincorporated areas where the migrants live. But these closely bunched bungalows have the cohesion of a neighborhood. North Nineteenth has more gardens than the sum total on Gardenia straight through Zinnia. Kept in a careless sort of fashion, they do not look manicured like the lawns on the opposite side of the tracks.

Dogs laze in front of the bungalows on patches of dried dirt, trying to rid themselves of fleas with their short legs. On the tiny porches, flowers and vines hang next to discarded iceboxes in a cozy collage of Mexicana. A dead end brings a narrow, densely populated street to an abrupt stop. An old freight car, the color of rust, appears in the back of a yard that was once the preserve of bustling trains—the end of the line, where locomotives leading the way had to be turned about as brakemen jumped off rungs to the tune of a blast, loading and unloading the produce and livestock en route to every part of the country. Locomotives that were home to the hobo who happened aboard are now huge trucks that traverse the country on interstate highways.

In the yard, dogs sniff the debris, stepping over empty bottles of Carta Blanca left behind by boys and girls in moments of abandon inspired by the terminal aura of the end of the line. Were the yard located in a more cosmopolitan spot, the "authentic" car would lend itself to conversion to a kitschy restaurant.

On North Nineteenth a reverent indifference to conversion reigns, as if the feelings of religion have been transferred onto the material world, inspiring a respect, even awe, for that which does not come out of the earth.

Julian is getting excited; we are nearing Maria Pineda's block. There is no hint of anything suspicious so far. The area, with its splashes of unexpected color, its hodgepodge housing and rusting old trains, is far more lively than the cluster of clinics surrounding the hospital.

The plan is to drive at a slow but inconspicuous rate past her house. Once we have some idea of what it looks like, we will park the car a few blocks away, and I will visit Maria Pineda. Julian balks; he wants to revise the plan and park the car at the corner so he can look out and see me in case I come running out of the house, behind me a mad Mexican with a butcher knife.

I suspect Julian has seen too many American movies. I am not afraid. I do not believe anyone will threaten my life, and if someone should, Julian's presence in a parked car at the corner would hardly be of help.

We slow down once we are on her block. We pass a tiny one-story church. LA ALIANZA, CHRISTIANA-MISIONERA reads a sign squeezed between two elongated trees, their shadows dwarfing the small adobelike structure.

Two doors away, a wooden bungalow sits on cinder blocks. The slats on the bottom third of the house and the trim around the windows and door are painted lavender. The top of the house is a tarpaper roof. There is no basement, but meters are visible on the side of the house. At least it has electricity and running water.

How are you going to question her, Julian wants to know. I am not sure. Maria Pineda is bound to suspect a stranger. From a jail in Houston, Jesse rang up Maria to say she had killed the woman he was planning to marry. Evangelina has also called and accused her of murder.

I will have to see what happens when we meet. It depends on how she responds to me. I don't even know if she is home. Driving past her house, I did not see any sign with a stork, like those I saw in the slides of *parteras* shown me by the sisters. A suspicious omission.

If she were only delivering babies, there would most likely be a sign. Otherwise, how would she get clients? I promise Julian to inquire about that, but he has other things on his mind. Find out where she got her training; how long she has been acting as a *partera;* what instruments she uses; whether or not she has a license to deliver babies.

I get out of the car and walk two blocks to Maria Pineda's. There is no bell. I open the unlocked screen door and knock once on the inside door. Through the transparent fabric that covers the glass, I can see straight to the back of the house. Several figures, all male, are moving in a room which appears to be a kitchen. Cots are strewn in an undefined middle room. Old appliances populate the yard as well as the back room.

I knock again. The figures move back and forth. Why is no one coming to the door? Are they quickly disposing of give-away details, or are they merely making coffee? Maybe it *isn't* safe to go inside. But the bicycle in front of the house and the sight of small children inside make the setting unconducive to crime. Despite previous fears, I am convinced that Mexican-Americans rarely murder Anglos; in fact, all evidence points to the contrary. And in cultures where *macho* runs amok, a crude chivalry often prevails with white women.

I give the door a more aggressive knock. A woman steps out of a room set at a right angle to the entrance. Behind her I glimpse a double bed. She holds up the flimsy fabric, takes a look at me, and then lets the curtain drop back. She seems undecided whether to open the door. I rattle the loose handle until it almost comes off.

"Can I speak with you, please?" To my surprise, the door opens. "Maria Pineda?"

She acknowledges her name with a quick nod. Although she looks frightened, fear does not seem her natural emotion. The plucked eyebrows, which form two widely inverted Vs over her dark eyes, give her face a defiant air. Her hair is covered with a short scarf tied behind her head, exposing large loop earrings. She is wearing a faded pink ribbed-cotton turtleneck top; it is too tight and pushes her full firm bosom upward where a swell of womanly flesh rises above the outlines of her pointed brassiere, making a sexy cushion for the rhinestone cross resting between her breasts.

Her wraparound cotton skirt falls above her knees, revealing hips no wider than her waist. Her legs are bare down to her gold slippers whose thongs are clasped firmly by crimson toenails. About forty-five, Maria Pineda could be a cosmetologist from Argentina; her get-up seems to have been inspired by pin-up pictures of Jane Russell and other American movie stars of the forties.

Were it not for the children playing inside, the house would not have a hint of maternity. Placing a hand on her hip, which sways upward and sideways as she shifts her weight, Maria Pineda holds onto the shaky doorknob with the other hand, exposing her many rings. Only her shifting eyes make her seem vulnerable.

"I am in trouble," I say, placing both my hands on my abdomen.

Maria's hands flail in the air as if to dismiss a strong irritant from her eyes. "No, no," she says.

"*Comprendo* English?"

Again she gestures with her hands while shaking her head sideways. A young child runs up to her, peeking out from behind her skirt, which he clutches as if in hiding. The men in the back take turns coming forward; after staring at me in silence, they return to the kitchen and commence speaking Spanish to one another.

"Come, we must have privacy," I say, walking into the room from which Maria emerged when I knocked at her door.

She follows docilely. Gently, I shoo the little boy away and close the door. On one side of the room is the double bed just barely visible from the doorway. Above it hangs a rug with Jesus stepping out from a sunset in a negligee. The religious motifs are coarsely woven with hot colors, making the rug a curious precursor to a psychedelic poster.

Maria sits on the lumpy cot opposite the double bed. I sit down next to her and whisper *"abortar."* Maria jumps up and runs over to a bureau, reaching for a mannequin's head resting on top. She rips off a wig and grabs a Bible hidden under the fake head of hair. *"Limpia, limpia,"* she screams at me.

"No comprendo."

"Clean," she says, wringing her hands with the motion used for washing. And then when I nod, she reverts to Spanish, repeating the word *limpia* while she crosses her chest.

There is a knock on the door. I open it slightly and motion to the man standing in front to go away. Maria now goes to the top drawer of the bureau. *"Baptista, Baptista,"* she cries, as she shoves a small object she has just removed into my hands. Calmly, I receive her offering—a cross about four inches high and two inches wide with tiny squares of mother-of-pearl pieced together and placed within the wooden frame. An iron body of Jesus has been pinned, literally, to the jewel-encased cross by two tiny nails hammered through each outstretched arm.

Sinuously submissive, the miniature Jesus mocks the hyped-up figure on the wall. With one leg raised slightly and bent inward at the thigh, and the drapery around the genitals as flimsy as Maria's curtains, the body looks like that of a beautiful young boy. Only the face is old, yet ageless, in the manner common to religious renderings.

Maria returns to the bureau and takes out a larger cross. "No," I say, as she attempts to hand it to me. I ask if there is someone who can act as translator. In broken English, she tells me to speak to the little boy.

I open the door; the men in the back seem frozen. Although I am only one and they are several, my Anglo skin gives me authority. I ask the little boy to find someone who speaks English and then, returning to the room where Maria is sitting on the cot with the Bible in her lap, I place the cross on top of the bureau and sit down next to her. When the door opens, a young woman enters with the little boy.

"Do you speak English?"

"Yes," she says shyly.

"Good. My name is Ellen and I need a translator. And yours?"

"I am Carmelita."

"And the little boy's?"

"I am José," he volunteers.

"Thank you, José, for finding Carmelita. Now you must leave the room so we can speak in privacy."

José doesn't move. Carmelita says something to him in Spanish, and, with his head down, he walks out at a sulky pace. For a moment, I am reminded of Julian.

The young woman, a neighbor, appears to be no more than sixteen. She learned to speak English in school and practices it at home by giving her mother lessons.

I tell her the procedure—I will speak to her and then we will stop every few sentences so she can translate what I am saying to Maria. If I am speaking too quickly, she must not hesitate to tell me to stop.

Carmelita nods.

"There is a woman who died after an abortion, and a friend who was with her at the time says she came here."

At the mention of abortion, Maria grabs the Bible from her lap and holds it up in the air.

"The government is sending down doctors to investigate the death, and they are going to visit Maria. We might be able to help her if she can give an account of what happened. The doctors are not interested in prosecuting Maria. They want to know what method she used. I'll stop here and you can tell her that."

Carmelita complies, speaking rapidly in Spanish. She must be getting the message across, for Maria protests loudly.

I tell Carmelita that it will look suspicious if Maria denies it. Saying no, no, no will get her into more trouble than if she tells the truth. (While I wait for my words to be translated, I have a sudden unpleasant recollection of Dr. Chester trying to elicit a confession from Rosie.)

Maria sticks to her story. Carmelita tells me she swears she never does abortions. Maria again becomes agitated when she hears the word *abortion,* and, holding up the Bible, moves closer to the edge of the bed. She glances toward the door, as if planning to bolt.

I drop the subject of abortion for a moment.

"Carmelita, ask Maria how long she has been a *partera.* "

"Twelve years, she says."

"Ah, twelve years," I say directly to Maria. She looks relieved. "Where did she first start working?"

"The Grasso Company."

"The Grasso Company?" I repeat, trying to figure out whether it is something medical.

Carmelita tells me it is on Twentieth Street, right here in town. "Do you know it?"

Carmelita shakes her head no. "Ask her what she did there."

"She says she packed shrimp."

I smile at Maria, who has stopped fidgeting.

"Where did she get her training?" Carmelita looks unsure. "Where did she get her *medical* training?"

"*Sí,* " Carmelita says, repeating the question in Spanish.

"Reynosa," Maria answers.

"Where in Reynosa?"

"She says in a hospital."

"How long did she work there?"

"A long time."

"Where is the hospital?"

"She doesn't remember."

"What did she do there?"

"She gave babies injections."

"What kind of injections does she give here?" It is the first time I have set up Maria. But she is alert and immediately says, "No injections." I do not press. It is going well, and I want to get all the information I can. Whatever discomfort I am feeling at tricking Maria into talking, I decide to ignore for the moment.

"Where do the women go when they want injections for abortions?" Maria stands up. "No, no. Not you, Maria. Tell her, Carmelita, I do not mean her. Also tell her that it is good practice for her to hear the questions. When the doctors come, they will ask the same ones, and it will be much harder to answer them if she has not heard them before. Tell her I know she didn't mean any harm. Tell her it happens. Things go wrong, even with doctors."

"She says she never does abortions."

"Ask her what injections the people in Reynosa give."

"*Carlequina,*" Carmelita says.

"Is that quinine?"

Carmelita looks uncertain.

"Do you understand?"

"Yes. I just don't know the answer. I mean I don't know the name of the drug."

"Ask her to say it for you slowly, then you can write it down for me the way you think it is spelled.

Carmelita nods. I hand her my notebook and she writes down c a r l e q u i n a. I drop the subject and move on.

"How long has she been working as a *partera?*"

"Twenty years."

"How long here?"

"Six years. She says she has been a licensed *partera* for twelve years."

"Ask her where her sign is. No, wait, ask her *if* she has a sign."

"She says she doesn't have a sign."

"Carmelita, do you know what the sign for a *partera* is?"

"Not really."

"Do you understand this conversation?"

Carmelita blushes. "Yes, I think so."

"If she doesn't have a sign, ask her how people know to come to her."

"She says she goes to their houses."

Maria is a shrewd woman. She is not going to give an inch. She thinks she has convinced me of her innocence. I have no desire to torture her; in fact, this is distinctly unpleasant. But it would be useful to know more about what she does in order to avoid future deaths.

"Tell her that the officials may be interested in teaching *parteras* better ways to make things sanitary so there are no more deaths." (The officials have not said that, but I intend to propose it to them.)

"She says she never does abortions."

"How long did she know Rosaura?"

This time she falls for my set-up and tells Carmelita she just knew her on the street, not in the house. I instruct Carmelita to pursue this line of questioning.

"Ask her how Maria knew Rosaura on the street."

"She asked for an abortion, but she told her she doesn't do it."

Maria is getting upset again. "Tell her *I* believe her, but there is a problem. Rosaura's friend says that Rosaura came here."

"No," Maria shrieks when Carmelita translates.

"Ask her how it is possible Rosaura's friend can describe the house and everything in it if she never came inside."

"Maybe she forgets whether she came inside."

There is something painful in outwitting Maria. And yet, I do not know how else to proceed unless she gives me the information. If she does, it is possible the doctors won't come to visit her, I explain to Carmelita. But if she doesn't, Maria may have to go to court to testify, and it could be serious. "A death, you know."

Carmelita looks concerned. She seems to trust me. I can see she is urging Maria to be honest. She wants to help her. I imagine she doesn't want the police in her neighborhood or the woman across the street on trial for murder.

"She keeps on saying she didn't do it," Carmelita says apologetically. "She says she never does it, that the girls go elsewhere."

"Ask her how many come to her for abortions."

"She says nobody comes. They know she won't do it."

Carmelita seems to detect the contradictions.

"Do you know if she does abortions?"

"No."

"Did you know about the death?"

"No."

Maria is beginning to move again, as if she senses the beginning of a conspiracy.

"Tell her it is okay. I will tell the doctors she did not do it."

Maria smiles. It is my first outright lie. I get up and put my arm around Carmelita.

"*Gracias,* you have been very helpful." I compliment her on her English and ask if she can stay a bit longer. She says sure. "The little boy, José, is he Maria's son?"

"No, he is her grandson."

"Perhaps I can meet the rest of the family."

Maria gives a shrug, and we follow her through the house. I observe two cots in the middle room. When we get to the kitchen, I look around for medical equipment, ignoring the men who turn silent, but I see nothing. There is a little shed behind the house which I want to check out. Lacking an excuse, I open the door and ask Maria to pose for a picture outside where it is light. Maria hesitates.

"Come, stand here," I say as I edge my way closer to the shed. "What is this?" I ask, poking my head inside.

The questioning over, Maria tries to be gracious; who knows, perhaps the Anglo reporter does want to help. "*Sientese, sientese,* " Maria says to the excited Doberman who tugs on his short leash as we step near his turf.

Without asking permission, I step inside the shed. On top of an old washing machine sits a potpourri of preservative mists—sprays for cleaning, sprays for keeping hair in place, and a spray for eliminating odor. It is hard to walk around without disturbing the clutter.

Pushing aside the frame of a folding chair, I move toward the back, drawn by large dots of lavender, aqua, baby blue, pink, and yellow. From a distance the coronas look like decorations for homemade cakes, the kind sold at church benefits. Next to the coronas, wrapped in a large cellophane covering, are white plastic flowers. In a bizarre association, I am reminded of the daisy chains worn by Vassar "girls" on graduation day. Behind the flowers are the stands for the Styrofoam crosses, delicate easels made of coat-hanger wire. Maria, the graveside cosmetologist.

"You made these yourself?" Maria nods proudly after Carmelita translates my question.

"For special times," the young woman adds. "They are, how do you say in English, corsages?"

Again, the daisy chain comes to mind along with proms; but the female rites of passage in the fifties did not include burials.

"Maria says you can take her picture if you'd like."

I snap a few shots as I conclude my tour. She may do her art work in the shed, but there is nothing to indicate she does abortions there. I decide she must perform that activity in the house. After I say goodbye to Maria and Carmelita, I try to pass the snarling dog with nonchalance. He pulls on his chain, but I make it to the front, where a green wooden pen serves as a makeshift container for two garbage pails, their lids askew. I photograph the pails with their overflowing bags of garbage, a photograph Julian would later use as part of his presentation on family planning at a medical conference held in Reynosa.

"God, where *were* you?" Julian says. "If it weren't for Mark, I would have come around to check up."

"Has it been that long?"

"Close to two hours," Julian says with a sigh of one unaccustomed to being kept waiting.

"Well, at least I'm still alive."

"Let's hear your report," Julian snaps back, impatient with banter. "How long before she admitted it?"

"She never admitted it."

"You must be kidding. I thought you were getting a tour of an operating suite."

"No, it was nothing like that."

"By gosh, don't keep us in suspense any longer."

"Okay. She denies she ever does abortions."

"Damn," says Julian.

"Let her talk," Mark urges.

"Look, it wasn't all in vain. First of all, we're lucky she was there. I now know how she looks and what her quarters are like. I even took some pictures for you."

"What's in the place?"

"I'll get to that in a minute. The point is, if we can get to speak with the woman who accompanied Rosie—Evangelina—we can ask her to describe the house, and we can compare what she says with what I saw."

Julian is not satisfied. He wants to know everything, step by step. But he is also worried. Maria might leave town; he proposes again that he go visit her.

I try to calm him. If anything, she is more relieved now. A stranger, a reporter from up North, questioned her and left, all smiling and friendly.

Julian cannot be calmed. "When can you get hold of Pauline?"

"She works every day except Thursdays and Sundays. I'll call her tonight."

"Can't you get her to take off tomorrow?"

"Come on, Julian," chides Mark. "She's not like us; she doesn't make her own hours. You just want to get a look at Pineda. Admit it."

"Of course I do. Do you know how frustrating it is sitting here with you in the car while Ellen . . ."

"While Ellen has all the fun," Mark finishes.

I propose we go someplace where we can get lunch, promising to give a detailed report of the visit.

Once comfortably seated by the pool of La Posada, we dial for room service on an outdoor house phone, and in the privacy of the enclosed patio I present a "protocol," borrowing from the vocabulary of professionals who are not accustomed to having a woman set the rules. I'll call Pauline to arrange a time for her to come to the hotel. I will meet with her alone. If Diane is free, she can join us. I will call to invite her over. She may enjoy seeing Pauline in a relaxed setting, away from her child.

After Pauline and I feel at ease with each other, I will introduce her to the doctors and they can speak with her, but if they plan to tape, they must secure her permission first. Assuming that all goes smoothly, I will ask Pauline to arrange for Evangelina to come over. This will involve delicacy and tact; her doctor has advised her not to cooperate.

I stress the importance of spending time informally with the women before any official inquiry. Mark is relieved not to have the responsibility of making contact with strange women. Julian is not but knows he has no choice and reluctantly agrees to go along.

EIGHT **PAULINE**

At exactly six o'clock the next evening there is a knock at the
door, announcing the appearance of a woman of surprisingly
generous proportions on the patio. It is Pauline, Rosie's intended
sister-in-law, the sister of Jesse, Rosie's fiancé. Her face is so
animated it is hard to think of her as middle-aged. It is difficult
to calculate the age of women whose appeal is not centered on
their gender.

Dressed in a comfortable rayon print dress and a navy sweater,
Pauline holds her spacious body as if it were a canopy covering
her toes which, in their pointed, low-heeled pumps, look tiny. Her
short black hair curls around her face in a softened version of a
pompadour. She wears no jewelry except for a gold wedding ring.

"I came here directly from work. I hope I'm not too late,"
Pauline says, standing at the entrance to the room, a round black
pouch pocketbook in her hand.

I invite her in and offer her a drink from the improvised bar.

Pauline requests a little of the coconut juice with just a touch
of vodka. I had asked her on the phone if she could come with
Evangelina, who witnessed Rosie's abortion.

"Evangelina cannot come tonight," Pauline says, taking a seat
on a baronial chair next to the large color TV. "Evangelina's
doctor keeps telling her it is not a good idea for her to talk about
Rosie. It might upset her too much. But I think I can work on
her. If I just go by her house and pick her up tomorrow after work,
I think she will come with me. Now that I have met you, I can
give her a report and she won't be so scared. Even I was scared

before I met you. But now I feel relieved," Pauline says, taking a sip of her drink. "You look so young and so . . . what is the word . . . hippie is what they would say down here. I like people who look like that. All the so-called hippies I know are the most tolerant people here."

I, too, am pleased by Pauline's surprising informality; on the phone she had sounded precise and businesslike. I tell her the doctors look even less like professionals than I do, or at least one of them does, and that I am certain they will be careful not to upset Evangelina.

"Good. She goes off so easily. It is the drugs they give her, I think. She is on strong medication, and she smokes too much grass. I tell her just one joint a night. I am not opposed to it; I just don't like to see her so confused. And she drinks too much. It isn't good for her. But I think she'll help. I'll try to see if she'll come tomorrow night." Pauline reaches for her glass on top of the TV.

I offer to get her some ice, grabbing a container which I take down to the machine at the end of the corridor. I scoop up the rounded cubes and rush back with the full bucket. I enter the room and notice the patio doors are ajar. Through the glass, I can see part of a print dress. When I step outside onto the patio Pauline is backed up against the outside wall, her drink in one hand, her pocketbook in the other. Julian is directly in front of her, his tape recorder already running. I hear him thanking her for coming. "This is a very important case to us," he says.

I am furious that he has violated the agreement we worked out ahead of time. He reminds me of the hungry media hound who ripped out Rosie's obit from the *McAllen Monitor.* In his haste to get his story, Julian has not even offered Pauline a chair. Even from a selfish point of view, he should know better: people do not open up when they are not at ease.

There are tears in Pauline's eyes, but he is willing to overlook them. Perhaps he regards her as a sentimental woman whose feelings he can dismiss in the name of science, of methodology, even though his behavior did not get him the information he wanted the first time he was in McAllen. I am seething but do not wish to further upset Pauline.

"Julian, I guess you've already met Pauline while I went to get some ice for her drink. Would you like one?"

"Not now, thanks. I'd like to speak with Pauline alone."

"Well, just for a few minutes, Julian, because Pauline and I were having a chat when I stepped out to get the ice."

I can hear the lilt of Julian's Australian accent as I walk away, leaving Pauline pinned against the wall.

Mark, Ward, and Diane are sitting in the only corner of the patio with any sun. It is the first time I have seen Diane since we spoke two weeks earlier. She has accepted my invitation to come over to enjoy the sun.

"He's such a tourist," Diane says of Mark, who is hacking away at a stubborn coconut. Today she looks like a movie actress, with her large sunglasses raised back on her hair and her perfectly fitted Continental-style denims and high-heeled sandals. Her spirit is much brighter than it was when she spoke of Rosie.

"Very jet-setty," I tease her.

"Well, at least I don't look like a tourist," she says, laughing at Mark's struggle.

Across the pool, some fifteen tall blond, Danish farmers in black suits, here to see the citrus farms, raise their cups in a toast. *"Skoal,"* they shout in unison. Retirees on the balconies wave to the farmers, and a waiter comes by with rum punch. It is the first time I have seen Ward take a drink. I take one, but cannot enjoy the festive mood.

"Where's Julian?" Mark asks.

I tell him that Julian is interrogating Pauline.

He puts down his knife. "I can't believe it. Not after all the C.R. work we had last night. Julian is like a child who has to be the first one on the scene when the fire engines arrive. He loves the adventure."

"Adventure," I say, my anger spilling out. "A hawk who descends on a hare likes adventure too."

Ward excuses himself for interrupting, but he must explain that Julian thought it would be more valid if he spoke to Pauline before I did. Although Ward doesn't say it, I suspect he believes the same thing.

Mark accuses Ward of being an apologist for the "male medical establishment."

When I tell him Pauline was not even offered a chair, Ward backs off. "It's time to stop Julian right now," he says, as if issuing a command.

"It's like a rape," Mark says, encouraged by Ward's authoritarian tone. I urge him not to exaggerate. Just go get Pauline and stop talking.

Mark asks me to go with him. When we return to the room, Pauline seems calm, and good manners prevail. We invite Julian and Pauline to join us in the corner of the patio.

"Hey, I'm getting wet," Julian cries out, as a group of boys volley with a ball, grabbing each other around the legs as they attempt to force each other's heads under water. "Who *are* they?" he asks indignantly.

Pauline explains they are local boys who do construction work.

Julian wipes his Indian shirt with a towel lying near his chair and proposes we all head for Sam's.

Mark asks how the rest of us feel.

Ward looks uncomfortable but doesn't protest. First he must make some calls. After he's finished, he'll drive us to Reynosa where we'll join Julian at Sam's.

"They look like a bunch of teen-agers out on the town, don't they?" I remark to Pauline as Julian whizzes by with Mark and Diane and we stand waiting for Ward in front of La Posada.

"He is very nice, that Julian."

"Good. I was a bit upset that he set out to interview you before we had a chance to talk."

"It wasn't that I minded. It was the way he spoke of Rosie. He referred to her as a case, but I can't think of her that way. I feel okay now. I didn't realize how late it is."

I decide to go get Ward. He is speaking on the phone when I knock and calls out that he will be down in a minute.

"I was just remembering how pretty this place was before they renovated it," Pauline says when I join her. "It was old and needed a paint job, but I preferred it. It's too synthetic now."

I catch myself being surprised at Pauline's sophistication and silently reproach myself. It makes me more impatient with Ward, as if his delay is another form of unconscious prejudice.

"How old are your children?" I ask Pauline, switching to light talk lest she sense what's on my mind.

They are twenty-two, seventeen, and nine, she tells me. Her boy, the seventeen-year-old, is sick with the flu. She should call him while she waits. As Pauline searches for a coin, I suggest she use the phone in my room while I go knock once again on Ward's door. I can hear him on the telephone, and I knock loud and hard.

"Just one more minute, please. I'll meet you downstairs."

"No, I'll wait right here," I snap back.

I do not hesitate to point out his rudeness after he hangs up. He, as well as Julian, has treated Pauline shabbily.

"Ellen, I am as upset as you at both my own rudeness and his. But my boss was on the phone, and I can't rush him off. In fact, I still have calls to make, but I don't want to keep Pauline waiting any longer. She is a remarkable woman. I have nothing but respect for her. I want to apologize immediately."

Had I known Ward was on the phone with his boss, I would not have been so angry. I ask Ward if he would rather not go out to dine.

Ward lights up. "If you really don't mind, that would be wonderful. But first, I must go down to apologize to Pauline."

I assure Ward I'll explain to Pauline. He can get back on the phone with his boss and we will take off for Reynosa ourselves. I envy Ward the luxury of being alone with his thoughts, doing his work. I, too, would like to retire to my room and sort out the day's impressions. A ride with a stranger is a strain; I am not looking forward to making small talk.

I tease Pauline that she could be a suburban matron with her station wagon, the first I've seen since I've been in McAllen.

"They're not common here, but it's very useful to have one. I go to a lot of meetings and I can give people rides home. In my neighborhood, I'm known as a radical. People say, 'Don't listen to her; she's a troublemaker.' Just because I speak out my mind. Like with the abortion issue. I used to be against abortion. Then when Rosie died, I changed my mind. I realized it is necessary for young women, although I still couldn't have one myself."

I am surprised and moved. It must be hard to be a "radical" alone. I wonder how "radical" I would be if I didn't have the support of my friends and family. Pauline, in her quiet, unassuming way, is an impresive woman. I chide myself for worrying about making small talk.

"The other mothers . . . oh, they think I'm a troublemaker, like I said. But they are very hypocritical. Some of them use the pill because they don't want any more children, but they tell their daughters that contraception is a sin. I don't believe in lying to children. I sit down with them, even my boy. There are no secrets. I think it best they know the truth. I tell my son if he is going to have sex with a girl, he must be prepared to assume some of the responsibility. And now, after Rosie, everyone in my family is very aware of the problem.

"See, most of the young women can't go out on dates, so they see their boyfriends in school. And then after high school, they marry. That is the only way to get out of the house. I think that is wrong. It doesn't give them a chance to decide what they want to do. I tell my children that there is nothing as beautiful as having a child if you want the child, and nothing as horrible as having it if you don't. And I know; I have seen it both ways."

Pauline acknowledges she is lucky. All her children were planned. She had them exactly when she wanted to.

"It's not impossible if you are careful," she says when I look surprised. "When my husband went back to school, I read about the rhythm method in one of his biology texts. If you use it properly, it works," she says. "But you have to be very careful. I keep a chart of my periods, and when I am in a danger zone, he withdraws. We have a joke: I call him Quick Draw McGraw. And I talk frankly with my children about birth control. I tell my daughters, if you're going to have intercourse, you should be prepared. It's best to love the man, I tell them, but I know it is not possible for most of them to wait for that—which is why I think they should use contraception."

As she continues to drive toward the border, she tells me about her oldest daughter who is in college. Pauline is concerned because her boyfriend is pressuring her to get married. "You know the men think if they sleep with a girl they own her. They call a girl by every name in the book. But what do they call themselves, I wonder."

Pauline becomes quiet; she seems to be meditating.

When she resumes talking, she says her daughter's friends secretly ask her for advice. They know she won't disapprove. "I try my best to help them. One who already has an illegitimate child needed a Pap smear, but she couldn't afford to pay for it. I told her to say she was going on the pill and that way she could get a battery of tests free."

It is easy to understand why Diane had once said, "She is like our mother." I wonder where Pauline learned so much. "You sound like the only social worker in the whole area."

"I wish I were."

I find her remark poignant, although it was spoken without self-pity. "Did you go to school?"

"No, I'm only a seamstress."

"It seems like such a waste. I can see you as a family-planning counselor. The young women trust you and feel free to open up with you."

"They do. I think I understand what they are going through. That's why I feel so bad about Rosie. I was just thinking about her a moment ago. If only she would have told me, I could have given her the money." Pauline reaches for a tissue.

"Why do you think she didn't?"

"She was ashamed. Because of Jesse she didn't want me to know she was sleeping with other men. She didn't feel right about doing it when he was in jail. I know she loved my brother; he was the first man who accepted her little girl. He has one too. Rosie sought affection through boyfriends. She was still looking for what she didn't get from home. Her parents handled it wrong when she was pregnant. They never let her out of the house. They didn't want people to see her.

"I think she felt alone when Jesse went to jail. But Rosie was very proud. She wouldn't go to her parents for a loan. She wouldn't ask her father for a dime, not after he kicked her out for being pregnant. What scared Rosie most of all was to raise another child alone.

"In case something happened to her, Rosie wanted her older sister to raise her little girl. She didn't want any more children until she found the right man and got married. She was trying desperately to be a good mother, but she also wanted to be somebody. I told her she could be both.

"But I knew it was hard for her because she didn't have any security growing up. I would say to her, 'Rosie, I respect myself. If you respect yourself, other people will respect you.' " Again, tears enter Pauline's eyes as she drives along the flatness; the farmstands empty of produce look forlorn silhouetted against the sky blown up with pink.

"Rosie was used by men too soon. I used to tell her, 'Rosie, take care of yourself. You are becoming a love junkie. Don't let men use you.' "

Pauline slows down the car. "I have to stop. I hadn't noticed the gas tank is nearly empty."

I say there is a gas station just before the International Bridge.

"Listen, do we have to go to Reynosa?" Pauline says in surprise.

For the first time it occurs to me that she doesn't really want to go. As with Ward, she was probably going along out of politeness. We don't have to go, I tell her and she, equally relieved of etiquette's burden, wastes no time in turning the car around.

"With my boy being sick, I don't want to get home too late."

I, too, want to return in order to see the Martin Luther King special on TV.

I am just in time. The King special is starting when I get back to the room.

I HAVE A DREAM. THAT SOMEDAY I CAN SIT DOWN WITH THE SONS
AND DAUGHERS OF THE RICH AND POOR, AND TOGETHER . . .

Moving as they are, I cannot concentrate on the familiar
phrases. It is Pauline's presence that is still with me. The utter
dignity of the woman, the ability to juggle paradox: "I could never
have an abortion, but for others it is necessary." My mind wand-
ers as I sit through the show.

TUNE IN TOMORROW FOR THE CONTINUATION OF THE LIFE OF
MARTIN LUTHER KING, and then the screen flips to a garter:
STRETCH YOUR MONEY, DIG FOR A DOLLAR.

MARTIN LUTHER KING. DIG FOR A DOLLAR. Pauline. Maria
Pineda. The contrasts evoke earlier scenes. A chaotic, dirty house-
hold, a dog on a chain, men lurking about a kitchen, a Bible
hidden under a mannequin's head, a tawdry tapestry all hooked
up.

"*Limpia, limpia; Baptista, Baptista.*"

"Stretch your bills."

A conscience covered by a wig merges with the calisthenics of
commerce as I fall off to sleep.

Later that night I am awakened by a commotion on the patio.
Julian has been detained at the border. His eyes were bloodshot
from too many *piña coladas* and too little sleep, and the border
guards became suspicious. They demanded to see his passport,
which he didn't have with him. It was back in his hotel room. He
protested. But the guards, looking at his long curly hair and silver
chains, did not let him cross back.

Mark, who has returned to find Julian's passport, invites me to
join them back at the border. It's really exciting, he says as I return
to bed.

NINE EVANGELINA

"Ah, look at this here. It's like a whole bar," says a chubby woman with thick glasses. Pauline introduces Evangelina, who is wearing peach pants and a gray T-shirt with a psychedelic emblem pressed on the front. Her body has the pudginess of a prepubescent girl who is frequently called "fatso."

"First I need a drink," she says to me. "I love to drink." Pauline suggests she hold off a while, but Evangelina insists she is a big girl who knows how to handle liquor. "Even if I don't, it feels good."

"Ooh, I like you," Evangelina says to me. "Please let me have a joint. I am so nervous."

"Perhaps afterward," I say, avoiding commitment.

"But I need one now."

Evangelina is sweating; her hand shakes as she lights a cigarette. I go to the drawer where I keep my grass.

"Evangelina, you promised me," Pauline says. "You know my son is going to come back to pick us up. I don't want him to see you stoned. He doesn't smoke yet."

Evangelina insists she must smoke in order to get through the interview. Pauline and I are in a bind: we want Evangelina to feel comfortable, but there is a sense that she is manipulating us. She knows she is the only witness to Rosie's abortion, the only one we know of who has seen Maria Pineda perform an illegal abortion. She may also be able to tell us if Rosie went to the *partera* because the Medicaid cutoff closed all other doors.

Noting the look of alarm on Pauline's face, I suggest Evangelina wait till afterward to smoke the joint.

She consents because she loves Pauline who is "the best person in the world," but if she doesn't smoke, she must have a drink.

"Evangelina, it is because I care for you that I tell you not to. It isn't good, not with the medication you are taking. I don't want to see you get sick. Remember the other time you passed out."

Evangelina gets up and goes to the bar, reminding Pauline that she is better now.

"Not too strong, Evangelina, please."

The telephone rings. It is Julian, wanting to know if Evangelina has arrived and when he can meet her. I promise that I'll call him when we are finished.

"Is that one of the doctors? Ooh, I want to meet him. Call him down now. Pauline says he's cute."

"They'll be down in a little while. Why don't we talk first? You, Pauline, and I. Then you can meet the doctors afterward."

"Can we go out dancing? I love to dance. And I love men, especially if they are cute." Evangelina sounds as if she has forgotten why she's here. As she pours herself a shot of vodka, Pauline again cautions her it is dangerous to mix alcohol with drugs.

I ask her what medication she's taking.

"Orange pills that make me real sleepy." I realize she's on Thorazine; it accounts for her slightly slurred speech.

We will never get started unless I become firm. I turn on the tape recorder and announce, "This is the story of Rosie's abortion as told by her friend, Evangelina." She takes a seat on the edge of the bed, and stares at the impromptu bar.

"Evangelina, what time did you and Rosie go there?"

Evangelina shakes her head, as if waking herself up.

"Let's see. Rosie came by Sunday at about seven-thirty in the evening. She had just been at a baby shower for her friend Roseann. She kept on begging me to take her to a woman who performs abortions. Now can I have another drink?"

"No, let's continue."

"I'm doing okay?"

"Yes, you're doing fine. Rosie said, 'Take me to a woman who does abortions,' and then what?"

"Then I took her to Maria Pineda's."

"How did you know to go there?"

"My mother told me about a woman who performs abortions. I called her and told her I need one for my friend."

"And then what?"

"She told us we had to pay her one hundred dollars in cash ahead of time and then come back later."

I am confused by her times. If they went at seven-thirty that night and had to come back later that evening, when did the abortion take place? I ask Evangelina if she can go back over the times.

"Ooh, I made a mistake. Can we start over?"

I tell her I don't want her to worry about mistakes. Whenever she remembers something different from what she has already said, she should stop the way she just did and start again. I assure her that nobody is using this as evidence about her.

"They're not? Oh, now I feel a lot better," she says, breathing heavily.

"Okay. So you went there and paid her one hundred in cash ahead of time. When was that?"

"About five-thirty."

"And what did you see?"

"There was another woman there. She looked very pregnant, about four or five months. You could really see her belly. Then she had an abortion and she walked out."

"Did you see the abortion?"

"No."

"How did you know she had it?"

"Because she didn't look pregnant anymore. I was going to have an abortion. I had gone to Maria Pineda's for a vitamin shot for one dollar. I was raped in the summertime and my daughter had run away from home and I didn't know where she was. I think she had run to her father's, but he wouldn't tell me."

Evangelina is going off. I do not point out that what she says sounds far-fetched. Better to get her to focus by asking a specific question about her daughter's age.

She says her daughter is fifteen and she is thirty, but she'll be thirty-one soon. And she has a son too. And did I know there was a little boy sleeping in Maria's house, Evangelina asks me.

Her associations remain loose, but at least we are back with Maria Pineda.

"Where was the boy sleeping?"

"At the *partera's* . . . Maria's. Even when Rosie had the abortion, the little boy stayed in the room."

"Did Rosie know the *partera?*"

"No, Rosie didn't know her. But the shots she had in Reynosa hadn't worked, and she was real desperate. That's why I took her. She kept on saying, 'I cannot have a baby. I already have one child and I want to take care of her right.' I could see she was really in a bad way."

"Okay. So you went back at seven-thirty. Is that right?"

"Yes, I think it was seven-thirty, or maybe seven. I can't remember. Maybe I should have another drink."

"No. The exact time doesn't matter. Let's go on. What happened once you were there?"

"Maria prepared all the instruments. She boiled them in a porcelain pot."

"What kind of instruments?"

"There was a rubber tube."

"About how long?"

"I can't do math. Maybe two feet."

"Two feet? This long?"

"No, not so long."

"Show me with your own hands."

Evangelina spreads her hands about twelve inches apart. "It looked like it belonged to a . . . what do you call those things you squeeze?"

"Douche bag?"

"Yes, that's it. Like for an enema."

"Where was Rosie?"

"In the bedroom."

At least it wasn't in the shed.

"What did the bedroom look like?"

"Well, it had a big double bed and a small cot."

"Can you remember anything else in the room?"

"There was a rug above the bed with a picture of Jesus."

"How did you see her boiling the instruments?"

"I made a mistake. I didn't see that. It wasn't very clean, but it wasn't my fault."

As Evangelina moves along with the story, her own guilt pours out. I try to help her by telling her that of course it wasn't her fault. Rosie was desperate and Evangelina didn't want to turn her down.

Again, Evangelina lets out a wheezy sigh. "I'm so glad you understand. All her friends stopped talking to me and I had a nervous breakdown afterwards and they had to put me in the hospital. My doctor said I shouldn't come here to talk about it because it might upset me too much."

I tell Evangelina how helpful it is she decided to come. Then I get back to the room in Maria Pineda's house. "So you saw this tube. A transparent tube?"

"I'm not sure. I remember Maria showed it to me afterwards. She said, 'I extracted blood from her.' I think it was a long red tube. Maria said Rosie was getting it real cheap. She held up a rag. The rag had blood all over it. It was an old rag."

"Was the rag separate?"

"No, it was tied around the tube, I think."

I hand her a napkin and a pen and ask her to pretend it's the tube and the rag. "It was like this," Evangelina says, as she drapes the linen napkin around the point of the pen.

"Did you see the procedure?"

"No."

"Where did you stay while it was being done?"

"Outside the bedroom."

"Can you describe it a little more?"

"Well, there is this . . . like hallway. Not exactly a hall, and after you walk in, there is the bedroom off to one side. Then there is another room with some cots. And in the back, there is a kitchen.

I waited in the room outside the bedroom where Rosie was."

"About how long was Rosie inside?"

"About half an hour."

"And then what?"

"Then Rosie came out."

"How did she seem?"

"She seemed okay."

"Was she in pain?"

"No. She said it didn't hurt. She said she was bleeding, but she seemed happy that it was over. She said she would do it again if she had to."

"So as far as you could tell, there was no sign that anything was wrong?"

"She seemed fine to me. Maria came out and said, 'I gave it to her real cheap.' And she told us it was guaranteed."

"And then what?"

"Then I drove to Rosie's apartment with my daughter."

"How was Rosie when she got home?"

"Rosie started to throw up at home. During the night Rosie got up and passed the embryo. My daughter stayed with her throughout."

"What do you mean?"

"Rosie called me and said, 'Evangelina, come over quick. My legs hurt a lot. They feel funny, like they're asleep.'"

"What time was that?"

"It was four-thirty in the morning. And I called Pauline."

"No, Evangelina," Pauline interrupts, "you mean four-thirty in the afternoon. Rosie went to school for the morning. She wasn't feeling well, but she did go to her class. She didn't begin to feel the ache in her legs till the afternoon."

"Oh, yeah, that's right. She said, 'Call my boss. I can't go to work.' She already had picked up Jenny from her day care and left her with someone. She didn't want Jenny to see her feeling so sick. I think she knew something was real wrong with her."

"So who went over?"

"Well, Margie went over to take care of her."

"Who's Margie?"

"She's this girlfriend who lived right near Rosie." I make a mental note to check out "Margie." "Margie won't talk to me because I took Rosie to Maria's. She thinks I killed her. When I went over in the afternoon, there was no one there, just an alley cat on Rosie's bed. The doors were wide open. And then I called Maria."

"Wait, I don't understand. You called Maria after you went over and found Rosie's apartment empty?"

"No. I called Maria one week after Rosie died. I told her, 'You killed my best friend.'"

"And what did she say?"

"She said, 'Come over and talk to me,' but I told her I have nothing to talk about. I said, 'I don't want you to perform any abortions.' That's all."

"I think she wanted to pay Evangelina some money," Pauline adds.

"Can I have my joint now?"

"You've done magnificently so far. Let's see if there is anything else."

"Oh, I just remembered something. Rosie said not to tell anyone. She didn't want Jesse to know she was pregnant. Also, it was a white tube, not red. I remember it didn't have any color because I could see the blood coming through it."

"How long did it all take?"

"About one hour."

"And Rosie, you say, was okay afterwards?"

"She looked okay, but she was weak. Mainly, she was relieved it was over. And I was glad it was over. Because I was raped in August and I needed an abortion and I was going to Maria."

"What happened?"

"I wasn't pregnant."

"Is Maria known in the neighborhood as someone who does abortions?"

"My mother knew her for that. About three or four years ago I knew someone who went to Maria for a shot."

"Did you see her use any injections?"

"No, just the tube and the rag. See, this is how it was . . . now

I remember real good." Evangelina picks up the napkin and wraps it around the pen. "Like this."

"You mean the rag was around the tube?"

"It was holding the tube. The funeral director said Rosie's body looked real bad, like a coat-hanger job. But I didn't do it."

Again I tell Evangelina that of course she didn't do it. I am moved by her. She has not come here to free herself of guilt; it is sheer will at work—an urgent need to prove that, despite the psychiatrist and Rosie's friends, despite the drugs and booze, she can get through this interview on her own.

Evangelina giggles with delight when I tell her she's done fine and that all she has to do is tell the doctors what she told me.

But she is now less keen on meeting them and wants to know why they can't just listen to the tape.

I try to explain that the doctors want to hear it for themselves, live. She is convinced it's because she wasn't good enough the first time.

Again, I say it has nothing to do with her. They would like to hear it for themselves; they think women can influence one another and feel it would be more scientific if they came and asked her the questions without me there.

"Please don't go," she begs. "I'm scared."

Pauline says she will stay in the room with her and that I won't leave until she feels at ease with the doctors. As I pick up the phone, Evangelina insists on another drink before they come.

"Easy, Evangelina. You don't want to be drunk for the doctors, and, more important, you don't want to make yourself sick," Pauline says gently but firmly.

Evangelina is still mixing a drink when there's a knock at the door.

Julian enters first, followed by Mark, as Ward holds the door open.

Julian sits on the floor by her feet, testing his tape recorder.

"Oh, he's cute," Evangelina coos. "Can I have a joint?"

"I really can't say," Julian answers, introducing himself. "Evangelina, we'd like to ask you a few questions. Ellen will return as soon as we're finished."

"But first a joint. Ellen knows where the grass is."

"Let me check to see if the tape is going. Are you comfortable?"

"Oh, you're so cute."

I close the door and temporarily retire to Mark's room. I am actually thankful for the break. All through the conversation, I'd had a desire to flee from Evangelina, like the rest of her friends. I suspect they have shunned her, not primarily for taking Rosie to the *partera,* but because they are frightened by her. Evangelina is a reminder of what they might become—a thirty-one-year-old mother without hope, plugged in, wired up with drugs and booze; a woman hospitalized for mental breakdown whose daughter has run away from home. Evangelina is too close to their own lives.

"Ooh, Ellen," Evangelina says when I return within a half-hour, "you didn't tell me how cute the doctors are. I like him, the one with the accent. He's so kind."

"She wasn't so good this time," Pauline whispers. "The joint. I knew I shouldn't have let her have it. She contradicted herself several times."

I tell Pauline not to worry—that there is no doubt the house she described is the same one I was in, and that is an important piece of evidence. The rest can be fuzzy. The doctors will have to piece together the details of the procedure from the hospital records. Pauline looks unconvinced.

"Look, it was wonderful you got her to come."

Julian is already talking restaurants. When he thanks Pauline and Evangelina for coming, I tell him to enjoy his meal and to take his passport with him if he's heading for the border again. After he leaves, I contemplate calling room service for the three of us who stay, but I want to split. It occurs to me that the entertainment in the Tesoro Club would provide a distraction and we could get dinner there too.

Evangelina wants to know if that's where the doctors are going. When I tell her I don't think so, she looks hurt. "I know they don't want to be with me anymore." This time I do not hesitate

to lie. "No, it's not that. They have work to discuss. They have
to be alone.

"I think we all deserve a break, don't you, Evangelina?" I say,
placing my arm around her waist. Her excess adipose makes her
body feel buttery. "You'll like it upstairs; there's live entertainment."

"Ah, all you wonderful folks, it's so good to be back in McAllen,
one of my all-time-favorite towns. I remember when Pop and I
would have drinks in St. Louis. Maybe some of you are familiar
with that divine little place. You all know about 'Meet Me in St.
Louis.' Well, darlings, they sang that for a reason. And to me, it's
'Meet Me in McAllen.' Pop and I always said if there's one town
we'd love to return to, it's that little town deep in the heart of
Texas. And here we are back again, Pop and me. Give him a hand,
won't you? That's it. And now, do any of you charming folks have
a request?"

" 'Feelings,' " Evangelina says softly.

"Did I hear 'Feelings?' " the singer says, and then breaks into
action.

Assuming the role of mother, I urge everyone to eat. But
Pauline stares at the shrimp creole.

"I don't have much of an appetite. I don't know why."

Evangelina leans over to speak to us, but this time her voice is
loud. "The best thing was for Rosie to die, if that was what was
meant to be. Don't you think, Pauline?"

TEN   A CASUAL REVELATION

It looks as if we are finished with "testimony," when Pauline produces a surprise witness. Roseann—a nineteen-year-old unwed mother who accompanied Rosie to Reynosa the day before Evangelina took her to Maria Pineda's—appears at the door with Pauline on her morning off.

Roseann, with a monumental face, is a cocoa-colored Montezuma of Mexican-Indian heritage. Sitting on the floor with her legs crossed and a shawl around her nylon parka, Roseann recalls every detail of the Saturday trip to Reynosa.

First Rosie washed the car and then she wanted a coconut drink without preservatives, but when she couldn't get it, she finally settled for a hot tamale, which she bought from a vendor at a corner.

Julian is impatient; while expressing an interest in the "human" side of Rosie, he does not want to hear what happened in between the car wash and the hot tamale—that Rosie stopped to order a cake for Roseann's baby shower. In medical school, future doctors are taught that a correct history follows a standard format. "This is the first admittance of a twenty-seven-year-old female of Hispanic descent whose primary complaint is . . ." The rhythm of question and answer should be staccato—to the point. Julian turns off his recorder as Roseann continues.

"I remember the woman said it was eight dollars. I told Rosie that was too much, but she ordered it anyway. 'I like this one because it says "Welcome Baby." ' I could see her mind was made up and there was no point to argue so I went with her to pick up the car from the car-wash place."

The next day, Sunday, Rosie had seemed her usual self at the baby shower—"real happy-go-lucky. It would have been impossible to know she had any troubles on her mind."

But on Monday, when Rosie didn't show up at the funeral home to pay her last respects to Roseann's mother, Roseann became suspicious. "It was not like her to just not show up. Rosie always kept her word. If she said she was going to do something, she did it. So I called her grandmother, who told me Rosie is in the hospital. She didn't tell me why, so I decided to visit her. 'Rosie, you look like the exorcist,' I said when I saw her. She had this reddish color, her lips were purple, and there was blood coming from her eyes."

Julian whispers to me that he has heard all this before. Can't I get her to be more concise, he asks.

But the weaving of tapestries with quotidian detail cannot be accelerated.

As Julian prepares to leave for lunch, he catches a reference Roseann makes to one of Rosie's previous abortions. Quickly he reaches for his tape recorder and asks Roseann to repeat what she has just said.

"I went with Rosie to Dr. Rivas when she told me she was worried because she had missed her period. 'I'm not going to let you go through another abortion if you are pregnant,' I say to her. I knew that she had once gone to Planned Parenthood because she told me I could go there and they would help me out with the baby."

"When did she go to Planned Parenthood?" Julian asks.

"I think she went to Planned Parenthood this past September," Roseann offers. "I know she went to Dr. Rivas and he gave her two shots in the breast."

"Yes, yes, I know about Dr. Rivas. That is all on the record. We also have confirmed that Rosie had an abortion in January 1977, in Harlingen." (This is news to me. The CDC team I am supposed to be working with, I learn, is not sharing information.)

Julian then asks about the 1975 abortion, the one Homer Rivas told *Ob.Gyn. News* took place in Mexico, a statement which has never been confirmed. "Do you know of any other abortion, and, if so, was it in Mexico?"

"You know," Pauline says after a moment, "I think Rosie did have another abortion. With a doctor here in McAllen."

"A doctor here in town? I don't believe it," Julian says, stunned. His shocked silence reminds me of my own reaction when Diane told me of Maria Pineda.

"Are you sure, Pauline?"

"Pretty sure. But you can check it."

Julian jumps up. He knows exactly where to check it. The only medical group in McAllen that performs abortions is Dan Chester's.

Chester's office confirms it. Pauline is right. Rosie's 1975 abortion did not take place in Mexico. It was right in McAllen, right in Dan Chester's office, and it was paid for by Medicaid.

Julian is relieved and proud. When feminists were screaming that women, poor or rich, do not seek out unsafe abortions, he did not cave in to contrary—and incorrect—charges by *Ob.Gyn. News* of "cover-up." *At no time did Rosaura Jimenez have an abortion in Mexico.*

Julian returns to La Posada dotty as a bird watcher who has spotted a baby egret. Nobody can argue with him any longer; he has it all—the proof, the evidence, the documentation straight from medical charts. Julian, Ward, Mark, the CDC, all are in the clear; it's *Ob.Gyn. News* that was wrong, just as he had suspected all along, he announces.

Mark is surprised that Dan Chester is the doctor who did one of the abortions. I am not only surprised, I am incensed. Julian cannot understand my indignation. I remind him that while Dan Chester hesitated to draw any connections between Rosie's death and lack of money, he did not hesitate to tell millions of viewers watching "Good Morning America" that Mexican-American "girls," such as the twenty-seven-year-old mother who died, seek out unsafe abortions for many reasons—shame, fear, a desire to keep a secret.

If Dan Chester had looked into his own files, he would have learned that when Rosie had the money she had no need for privacy. She went directly to Dan Chester, who also had no hesitation about the abortion when there was money.

Only when there was no more Medicaid did Rosie go to an untrained person, knowing that the laws of the womb do not change to accommodate Congress. When lawmakers vote that poor women must carry their pregnancies to term, the cells are not granted the power to veto. The fertilized egg divides into two whether Homer is in town or isn't; the divided egg turns into a blastula whether Dan Chester does an abortion or doesn't; the blastula becomes a gastrula even if Raphael Garza thinks *all* abortions are criminal acts. Which leaves women no choice but the Maria Pinedas who terminate pregnancies before it is too late.

Chester, Carter, and Califano do not like to see a woman die; even a single death is one too many, especially if it is as unexpected as the protoplasm that persists in dividing; as unexpected as the infection that continues to spread, slowly breaking down the vessels, starting with the larger and winding up with the tiny capillaries that spilled forth blood from Rosie's eyes as if she were some medieval martyr.

Julian tries to make excuses for Dan. Not even the best of doctors can be expected to remember the names of all their patients. I cannot accept Julian's apologies. Dan Chester triggered the investigation, and he knew from the start that Rosie's prior Medicaid abortion history was crucial. He should have checked his records. In his files was the information that would have prevented the backlash and subsequent confusion. It was also in Lila Burns's files. Did no one at CDC think to check those files? What kind of investigative team was this?

Julian says I am not being fair. Come on, do you remember the name of every student you have ever taught, he asks. I admit I do not. But Julian, I yell, were I asked to address the nation about the death of one, I certainly hope I'd have the sense to see if it were someone I knew, especially if what I was telling millions of Americans was also going to influence government policy.

It is hopeless; Julian insists that Dan Chester did everything "humanly possible under the circumstances." Julian has a tennis date with Dan, and after the game he and Mark have been invited to his house for cocktails. But Mark and Julian are split; Mark thinks it grotesque that Dan didn't know he performed an abortion on Rosie.

I ask Julian where Dan lives. Julian wants to know why. To take a picture of his house, I say, and put it next to one of Rosie's grave and inscribe the coupling with Dan's own words: "Theoretically there could exist a woman who cannot afford an abortion." And I'll underline the *theoretically.*

Julian will have no part in embarrassing Dan. "It's not just Dan. It's the whole damned profession," Mark blurts. In an aside he says to me, "I don't know exactly which streets you take, but it's this modern place with huge redwood trees and a two-story cathedral window from which you look out at this garden."

We are all seated in my room on beds and the floor; Mark is trying to explain to Julian about cronyism when a short dark man with a mustache and an attaché case appears at the patio door. It is Mark's boss, Dr. Stanley Music. He opens the door, steps into the room, and announces that he has heard about the "goings on" in McAllen while on assignment in Korea. It seems the top officers at CDC have become nervous about the investigation. They are uncomfortable that, during the taping of Evangelina, three male doctors were with two Hispanic women and no outside witnesses were present during the proceedings. Suppose the women accuse the doctors of rape? How will they deny it? But, Dr. Music says, what got him was the news that "his boys" had documented one of the previous Medicaid abortions done on the dead woman prior to the fatal one. It was *that* that made him decide to fly directly from Korea to McAllen en route to Atlanta.

Dr. Music scrutinizes the scene; it is apparent he does not see before him a serious investigative team. Focusing attention on my long peasant skirt, he asks, "And what are you doing down here?"

"Working on a story. And yourself?"

Dr. Music hands me a card from his attaché case. On it is printed his name, followed by letters signifying numerous degrees.

"This doesn't say anything about why you are here," I comment as I put the card aside and he takes a seat.

"Have you ever heard of a disease called smallpox?" Dr. Music asks. Then, without waiting for an answer, he places his hands on his knees and lectures on the history of the disease, concluding, "This is the first year there has not been a single case recorded throughout the world."

I ask Dr. Music if he really believes I have not heard of smallpox. "Of course not," he says. "I was merely using the well-known device of starting out with a rhetorical question. As a writer, you surely have heard of *that,*" he says before launching into a lecture about "the necessity of using accredited means" when it comes to publishing the truth.

"I hate to interrupt," Julian says. "But I must report to you, Stan, that we can now publish an updated story in the *MMWR.* We have proof not only of the Harlingen abortion done in 1977 with Medicaid money, but today I found out about another Medicaid abortion done here in McAllen." Julian does not say by whom.

"You mean, we triumphed over *Ob.Gyn. News,*" Dr. Music says, sounding so pleased that he momentarily forgets about accredited means.

And Julian hands me a draft of the report they have been working on. Although it's rough, he is proud. "And you, Ellen, ought to be damned pleased. You're going to be listed as the primary reporter on an *MMWR* article."

ELEVEN

CONFRONTATION WITH HOMER

Texas was built in the superlative. According to the *Tomlinson Lone Star Book of Records* I bought at the Houston airport, South Padre Island is the longest seashore in the United States, with a barrier reef that stretches one hundred and ten miles. The compilers of the book should take a look at the motels at South Padre Island. Memory Motel, Sun and Sound, the Merry Mermaid, Rod and Reel—perhaps the most motels with alliterative names bunched up in the shortest space. Beachcomber, Honeymooner, No-Tel Motel could be entered under "greatest expectations."

Homer suggested I head out to South Padre Island in a phone call I made to him while the CDC doctors were preparing their updated report. It was early when I reached him in his office, and he was surprised to hear from me. "Let's get together."

"What for?" he asked teasingly.

"You'll see."

Homer agreed to meet at the hotel at the end of the day after dinner. To keep the conversation light and civil, I asked him if there were any sightseeing spots he recommended I visit during the day. He suggested South Padre Island. "It was one of Rosie's favorite getaways, and I think you'll like it too."

I can't easily imagine a platonic friendship between the two, but perhaps they confided in each other. According to Roseann,

Rosie trusted Dr. Rivas. "He never made her feel funny like the other doctors did."

I can see each sifting the other's vulnerability through romantic strainers. Approaching the bridge that dips graceful as a tern, I begin to feel the tug of yearning. It is easy to imagine Rosie and Homer confiding about lovers who have spurned them. Physically small, ethnically insecure, and filled with dreams of escape, both Homer and Rosie were drawn to what passes for hip in South Texas.

The square boxes built of glass that levitate from the sand, with the aid of wooden beams, are surrounded by bungalows that predate the rash designs of instant resorts.

Everywhere is expectation.

Freed from concern with "accredited means," I indulge in the corny melancholy inspired by the sea, recalling every road not taken, as dusk approaches.

Later, on my way back to La Posada, I stop at Pelican's Wharf, in the center of the Family Shopping Mall. Homer recommended it the first time we met. I am hungry and there is a certain symmetry to concluding my sightseeing at South Padre with Homer's initial recommendation.

Pelican's Wharf is bordered by a wooden deck with ropes strung along posts. In the lounge a young man with a red beard strums a guitar and sings a song about lonesome cowboys.

A young man with a Boston accent seats me in the dining section and then introduces me to the dining procedure like a solicitous upperclassman on the first day of school. After I have mastered the various stages of dining, we chat about things up North. A fairly new arrival, he has come down to join some friends of his who dropped out of college to open a restaurant.

I order a drink from the bar person and then am invited to help myself to salad. The cauliflower, carrots, beans, cucumbers, and diced onions are all fresh; so is the bread, which is warm to the touch. Back at the dining booth, there is a young woman prepared to take an order for wine. A large piece of parchment paper that looks like a medieval telegram is the menu.

The man with the Boston accent returns, vouching for the

freshness of the catch of the day—red fish. "I picked it up early this morning after it came in from the Gulf. It's real good. I have an idea you'll like it," he says, implying that red fish goes with my character.

At the fourth inquiry to see if there is anything I would like, I say I would like them to stop asking. "No sweat, man. I got it. Enjoy your meal and hope to see you again real soon."

The excessive concern of the staff is incongruous with faces that resemble those of forest rangers rather than those who have spent a lifetime waiting on others and have adopted affability because their livelihood depends on it. At Pelican's Wharf, the solicitousness does not feel calculated; rather it seems to reflect the culture of south Texas. Pelican's Wharf, situated so aptly in a shopping center, could serve as a symbol for fake roots—the link between Rosie, Homer, and their strivings to escape their Mexican heritage, only to wind up migrants among benignly synthetic landscapes.

At 8:00, Homer, in a denim jumpsuit, knocks on the patio door. Before opening it, I switch on a tape recorder hidden in a bag on the bed.

"You never did send me an autographed copy of your book," Homer says as he stares at himself in front of the large unframed mirror. "Of course, I read it long before I ever met you," he adds, looking over his slim small figure and pulling on his sideburns. Although many self-proclaimed male feminists have lots of hair, I've often suspected that most secretly yearn to be tall and good looking in an all-American kind of way.

"Are you putting me in your latest book?" Homer inquires.

Abruptly, I switch to Rosie. "Why didn't you do something to help her ahead of time?"

"I was not available when she had the abortion. I told you that already."

I do not let Homer get away so easily; I know a lot more now than when we first spoke. "You knew her history; you knew she had several unwanted pregnancies. I want to know why you didn't do something when Rosie told you she missed her period and might be pregnant."

After announcing "I'm not an abortionist," Homer recalls a childhood incident. "When I was a little boy my mother took me to the doctor for an ingrown toenail. The doctor made me strip. When I was standing totally naked, he pulled on me to get some fluid. He was trying to see if I had VD. I never forgot it. I determined that one day when I became a doctor I would never do unnecessary VD testing to anyone. Especially Rosie."

I do not bother to point out that we are not talking about VD, for I know that once male feminists get going on a confessional binge, they will reveal every last humiliation with pride—how they first wet their bed, shit in their pants, had a bout of impotence. The male feminist seems to confuse humiliation with sensitivity.

"Homer, why did you tell the reporter from *Ob.Gyn. News* that if Rosie had come to you ahead of time, you would have done something to help her? Rosie *did* come to you ahead of time. Twice."

Aware that he is caught in a lie, Homer turns. "You're not a doctor. I don't have to talk to you."

"True. Would you be willing to talk to a doctor?"

"Sure, any time."

"Good. The doctors from the CDC are here at La Posada. You can talk to them immediately."

"I'm not talking to anyone tonight."

"So you won't talk to me and you won't talk to the doctors. Okay then, please leave."

Although he has had his hand on the doorknob, Homer hesitates. "I'm going to call my lawyer," he announces, unexpectedly.

"That's a good idea," I say, adding that I, too, am going to speak with lawyers. I want to discuss from a legal point of view why Rosie's personal physician ignored her complaints. Homer looks genuinely alarmed.

"I'm a very busy man. I can't go checking out every complaint. Besides, I did treat her."

"For a chest condition. What you did find time to do is speak with reporters. In addition to saying that you would have treated Rosie had she come to you ahead of time, you even went so far as to say that you knew *for a fact* that Rosie did not use Medicaid funds for her 1975 abortion when they were still available. Another outright lie."

Homer tries to defend himself. "There can be many versions of the truth," he says philosophically.

"Not in this instance," I tell him.

Homer begins to fidget with his jumpsuit zipper. I tell him that I do not want to waste any more of my time.

"Your time," he counters with unexpected authority. "I'm the one who is the doctor."

TWELVE **MARGIE**

The houses of Colonia Hermosa are hard to distinguish from the outhouses behind them. The pickup trucks parked in front are larger than both. I comment to Pauline that in less than a decade Rosie went from an outhouse to a college classroom.

"The younger women don't want to be used the way their mothers were," Pauline says. "I think the drugs may help the sex. I gather there isn't the same rush. The girls tell me they like it when sex is slow; it gives them more pleasure. To me, what's most important about drugs is they have shown the girls that they needn't have sex only if they want to have children. Most of the young girls get on the pill as soon as they can."

As we drive slowly down the dirt road, little children stare at us. Their stomachs are bloated. How mixed is the bounty of the land where children who gather citrus fruits walk around with parasites in their intestines because there is no potable water to drink. It is clear why the women get on the pill as soon as they can. And learn how to drive cars. They do not want to spend a lifetime stooping over—planting, picking, and being fertilized all in a single day—on borrowed land where spoilage and genesis remain intertwined.

Once past the *colonia,* Pauline points to a new brick building. Its aluminum cross is as sleek as the nose of the Concorde. A complicated set of arrows, blinking lights, and other engineering niceties direct the flow of traffic from the main drag into the parking lot. It's the church where Rosie was going for counseling —the church of Calvary Baptist. They held her funeral service there, Pauline tells me. The pews look as functional as a set of avocado-colored kitchen cabinets.

There is one person left to speak to—Margie. Like Diane, she lives in the garden complex. Like Diane and Rosie, she is unmarried, has gone back to college, and is raising a hyperactive child.

"Okay, now sit down," Margie says to a little boy who is standing rubbing his eyes. "This is a new friend," she adds, pointing to me. "Come on, you know Pauline. Here, eat this," Margie says, gently but firmly, slipping a plate with French toast onto the table.

"No," he screams out.

"Okay, you don't have to sit with grownups if you don't want to. Come sit in your high chair if that's what you want. I'll let you eat there just this once."

The little boy obediently follows his mother and the plate of French toast, settling into a chair behind the aqua counter, among the kitchen appliances. Margie goes to pour some milk from a large carton and then joins us at the table.

She offers a striking contrast to Diane; there is none of her softness. Margie is direct in speech, almost brusque. Her clothes, too, are different—shorts, T-shirt, walking shoes. Her hair, combed back, reveals a serious face. There is no nonsense to Margie.

Pauline has already spoken with her to explain our visit. Margie says she's surprised I didn't come to talk with her the first time I was in McAllen. "I found out about the investigation from Diane," she says and begins.

"I remember on Monday before Rosie got sick, we went to school together because we both had a class in government. She said to me, 'Let's have a bite to eat. I'm going to skip the next class.' Now Rosie never did that, so I was surprised. She said she wanted to talk.

" 'I love Jesse and really want him. I don't want to go out on him. It's just something I have to do.'

" 'No, you don't,' I told her. 'Just blow these other dudes.'

" 'Margie,' she says, 'don't judge me bad. It's something I have to do. We're going to end up getting married. I want to make sure it's right before we do it. I'm going to tell you something, but don't get mad at me. I think I'm pregnant.'

" 'Goddamn, Rosie, of all things.'

" 'I couldn't help myself. See, I knew that it wasn't Jesse's.'

" 'What are you going to do?'

" 'That's just it. I don't know. Planned Parenthood is not going to pay for it.'

"I was really pissed with her. I mean she had everything going. Rosie was real smart. She was a good student and she was almost ready to graduate. I couldn't understand why she would go and get herself pregnant. I know we all did it, but we stopped.

" 'You aren't going to get anywhere unless you can manage on your own,' I told her. 'You can't trust men to do it for you. That much I know.'

"When I started messing around, I was living with my mother on welfare. At fifteen, I became pregnant. I didn't want my mom to know. Mexican mothers are not that liberal. She didn't want me messing around. I was very young. I don't know why, but I ended up talking to my boyfriend about it. He told me that for forty dollars I could go to Reynosa. I was just walking around and I ran into a friend. I explained why I was in Reynosa and she said she would come with me. The office was filthy, but I went ahead anyway. I didn't care. I didn't want a child. They told me it was the Foley method.

"I came home afterwards and I was sick, hemorrhaging. I told my mom that it was just my period. 'Mom, don't be scared.' I acted real cool, but I was dying. I mean I was getting cramps the whole week.

"Then a year later I got pregnant again. I didn't know anything about the pill then. So I went to a pharmacist lady in the back of the store in Reynosa. That was dirty too. She inserted a tube in me and left it in and told me to return in twenty-four hours so she could remove the tube. I returned and I was fine. I even took off and went to a concert that night.

"The next year when I got pregnant I went to Dr. Chester.

Now abortion is legal, I thought; why go to those filthy joints. All you need is a little over two hundred bucks in cash. Chester was real good. He said as soon as he finished, you're ready to play football again. He didn't even give me anesthesia. That's how easy it was. That was 1973.

"In 1974, I was three months pregnant and the doctor said to me, 'Why do you want another abortion?' And I thought about the question. 'I'm paying off a car, and I don't have a husband,' I told him. 'Well, there's always welfare,' he said, and gave me the number of several agencies. I figured it was time I stopped being a wild person like I used to be. I was twenty-three, you know. I wasn't a kid anymore. And so I decided to have the child.

"Now I'll get stoned, drunk, play around, but when it comes to the nitty-gritty, I don't do it so fast. After Joey was born, I got on the pill. By now I knew that when the man says, 'I'll take the responsibility,' don't believe him. I used to think when I was young that he meant he'll marry me and help support the baby if I get pregnant. Then Rosie told me that he means he'll pull out. But when it comes time to actually doing it, I discovered he doesn't even mean that.

"Rosie was real smart. If it hadn't been for her, I wouldn't even be in college. She got me and Diane to go, you know. Anyway, I didn't see Rosie after that Monday in school. Then Sunday night I got this call. 'Guess what?' Rosie says. 'I don't think I'm pregnant.'

"I figure she miscalculated her period because she wasn't that regular. She was on the pill one month and off the next. She kept on alternating because she thought it would be better for her system. She was a health nut. She used to get her food in the health store and she worried all the time about her health. So I told her I was real glad that she wasn't pregnant and that maybe this scare would put some sense in her head.

"And then the next day, Monday, I was home by one o'clock. My phone was out of order. So I went over to Rosie's. We always went into each other's place if we had any problem. I was about to say, 'What are you doing here at this hour?' but she was asleep and I didn't want to disturb her. A little later I had to use the phone again. She was still asleep, but now the cover was on the floor and she wasn't wearing any clothes. I could hear her moaning. 'Are you all right, Rosie?' I asked. She sort of nodded and mumbled something about trouble with her period. I figured it was bad cramps and that's why she was moaning. I had to pick up Joey at four.

"I got back and we were eating supper when there is this knock on my door. It's Rosie's boss. 'Who's Rosie's doctor?' he is asking. 'She's very sick. We have to call him.'

"I went right over. I was going to check in with her after I fed Joey anyway. I see Rosie. She's all cramped up. 'Please take me to the emergency room,' she is saying. 'Hurry. Hurry.' I rush back and grab my kid. 'Come on, let's go.' And I lock up my house and go back to Rosie's.

"The man next door has to help carry her out. It took the two of them to get her off the bed, and that's when I notice blood on the sheet. She had told me before she was having trouble with her periods. 'Rosie, are you hemorrhaging?' I asked. And she says yes. Now I'm getting real scared. Every time I hit a bump I can hear her scream. I have no idea of what is wrong. It doesn't seem like just cramps from your period. I'm really racing to get to the hospital. 'Give me your Medicaid card, Rosie, so we don't waste any time when we get there.' But she doesn't move. Her boss is in the car behind us with my little boy. I'm driving while I'm trying to look for it.

"When we pull up to the hospital, I see this chick is really sick. She's purple beneath the eyes. 'What's wrong with you, Rosie?' 'I can't feel my legs,' she keeps on saying. 'Come on. Let's hurry up,' I call out to the guys to get the stretcher ready.

"Once she's on it and being wheeled inside, I tell the nurse she's bleeding from her insides because that's all I know. Then I get my little boy. I feel relieved. At least we got her to the hospital. I figure they'll take care of her. She's going to be okay once they stop the bleeding. Thank God we got her there in time. And I'm real glad that I was home to be able to drive her.

"I go in to check on her before heading back. God, did she look terrible. By now Pauline is there. Where's Jenny? Pauline tells me the grandma has her. I'll get her, I say.

"I come back home and call the grandma up. I tell her I think Rosie is having a miscarriage and that she's in the hospital. I tell her I have Rosie's purse. Rosie had said to take good care of it because it has her scholarship check in it. Her grandma says she'll come by to pick up the purse. So I go next door to lock up her apartment. It was real weird, man, there's just this stray cat sitting on her bed. We were in such a rush I guess we left the doors wide open.

" 'How's Rosie?' I ask when her grandma comes by. 'The doctors don't assure her life,' she says. '*What?*' And then I just freaked out.

"That Sunday night when she called me to tell me she wasn't pregnant, I thought everything was all right. She was complaining a little, but I thought that now she's not pregnant, she is going to find something else to worry about. So I just blew her off because she was a hypochondriac. Then I find out that Rosie took four Darvon on Monday in her government class to kill the pain. She left the room to take the pills. That's what Diane told me afterwards. But Rosie couldn't tell me. See, I had already changed. She was embarrassed. I kept on telling her don't hang out with bad people. Don't hang out with Evangelina. It will influence you.

"She got out of her government class by twelve-thirty and went straight home. Blew off work. She called in to her boss to say she was sick. Then she went to sleep. That's when I found her in bed. Even though she must have felt real sick, she didn't forget about Jenny. She called a cousin, a guy who works at the hospital as an orderly, in fact. She told him to go pick up Jenny at the day-care center and take her to the grandma's. See, she had it all arranged so Jenny wouldn't see her sick. I have the feeling her boss knew she had an abortion; otherwise, I don't see how he would have known to get over, how he would have known she wasn't fooling, that she was really sick.

"When she was working, she met this guy who worked next

door at this head shop, and she was messing around with him. She always had a weakness for a rich boy. And he was good looking. But I say, hell, they're all the same, rich or poor. They just want a piece of ass, no matter what they look like or how much money they have, and if you get in trouble, forget it. They don't want to know you.

"I think it was her boss who gave her the money for the abortion. I heard on TV that the reason she went to have an abortion in Mexico was because she was embarrassed. That's a bunch of bull. Just money. All the time it was just money. Rosie was such a unique person. She had it all together. She had always been on her own since the time they threw her out on the streets. If you needed money, you can borrow it, she'd say. She got me by the hand and took me to school. She explained how to get government loans. That's why I'm so grateful to Rosie. Money was always a problem, but whatever she had, she shared. And she kept up a good front, even when she was scared herself.

"Like this check that was in her bag for seven hundred dollars. It was her scholarship money. That was sacred. She wouldn't use it for anything, except maybe to feed Jenny if she had to. But she always gave Jenny the best and she wasn't going to cash that, not even when her food stamps were robbed.

"When her family came down from Houston, they were all fighting over the money. They wanted to cash it before she died. I guess they thought it might not be good after her death. Rosie hadn't even tried to cash it for the abortion. That's how much school meant to her. And she had big expenses because Jenny is a hyperactive little girl. Right, Pauline?"

"Yes. I stayed with her for the three days Rosie was in the funeral home. Jenny screamed so hard when she saw Rosie in the coffin I thought she would lose her voice. I tried to take her out to the playground, but she wanted to be with her mother. Rosie looked like a little rag doll, even though they put her in a white dress. I guess she would have worn it if she married my brother.

"I didn't tell Jesse the truth when Rosie died. He had enough loss. Security in a child growing up has a lot to do with things. Jesse and Rosie were alike. They were both seeking affection and they were both a little bit lost. I think that's why Rosie started seeing a pastor. It was like counseling. She wanted to change, I think . . ." Pauline takes out a tissue. Her large regal body begins to tremble.

"I keep thinking if I had been there for Rosie to talk to she would still be around today. Where did I go wrong, I ask myself."

"You didn't go wrong anywhere," Margie says to Pauline. "It's just one of those accidents. Rosie could never have come to you. It's not your fault you're Jesse's sister."

"But she spoke to the pastor," Pauline protests, and then begins to sob. Margie hands her a tissue. It is the first time I have seen Pauline break down.

After a few minutes, Margie resumes. "Look at it this way, Pauline. With so many investigations, it's like she's not really dead. Rosie's going national."

PART 3

TAKING ACTION

THIRTEEN **THE ARREST**

I returned to McAllen in June. This time with Frances Kissling, who was eager to meet Diane and Pauline. She had heard so much about them since that day in October when she had first told me of Rosie's death.

Frances also had specific things on her mind: to plan a memorial fund in Rosie's name and to clarify some questions about another complication. She had promised her colleague, Dr. Julian Gold, that she would try to find another Mexican-American woman named Marta, whom Dan Chester had turned away, to obtain details of the illegal abortion that led to her bout with tetanus. The information could help the CDC determine if the abortion had been performed by Maria Pineda. Mark and Julian were easily put off when Marta was not home. They left their number but Marta never called back.

Frances and I were both curious to know the results of the February investigation. As had happened many times before, we quickly became immersed in rehashing the details of Rosie's death and the investigation—a useful if tedious process.

My relating the interview with Maria Pineda led Frances to speculate: What had happened to Maria Pineda since she was visited by me and then by the CDC? Had the CDC reported her to anyone? Were the police called? In fact, why was there not a police investigation at the time of Rosie's death? *Should* there have been a police investigation?

That evening I called Pauline, who came by immediately. We expressed to her our concern about Maria. Pauline voiced her sense of helplessness: Maria Pineda was still free to practice, no one really cared about Rosie's death, and, despite our efforts, nothing in McAllen had changed.

Perhaps, she felt, the authorities needed more evidence. How could we prove beyond any doubt that Maria Pineda was still doing abortions?

Pauline then suggested: "Diane and I could go to her as a mother and daughter. I will try to convince her to give Diane, 'my daughter,' an abortion. I'll tell her that my husband will kick her out if he finds out she is pregnant."

We moved quickly, enlisted Diane's help, then drove right to Maria Pineda's house. Frances and I waited about half a block away, sitting quietly in the car and a little bit afraid for Diane and Pauline. What if Maria became suspicious or recognized one of them as a friend of Rosie's? I sympathized with Julian's earlier impatience at being left waiting while I had interviewed Maria.

After what seemed an eternity they returned, Pauline beaming, Diane drawn and frightened. Maria Pineda believed them. For $125 she was willing to help Diane as she had helped Rosie in September 1977. Her work was guaranteed.

Pauline told of the scene in Maria's house, of small children and their mothers. Several children had sores on their legs and were receiving penicillin injections from Maria. Pauline was also told by Maria that she had just done an abortion for another woman.

Now Pauline and Diane were even more willing to continue. But Pauline, with children of her own in the neighborhood, could not risk possible retaliation. She promised to find Marta and gain her cooperation. Diane, who now saw some way of making sure Rosie did not die in vain, would return for the abortion.

Thoroughly exhausted, but hopeful of finally getting action, we separated for the night. Pauline agreed to come by the next evening with Marta. Diane, who was enrolled in summer school, would plan her story for Maria and be ready after classes. Frances and I said we would secure government help—we were, after all, colleagues and co-investigators with the CDC team.

* * *

Thursday morning, June 8, 1978, we began our work early. It was one of the most discouraging and disillusioning days of the investigation.

We called Julian Gold at the CDC, who told us that he, too, had received confirmation that Maria Pineda was still performing abortions. Just three days earlier, Marta, independently of our work, had finally reached him. While she denied that her abortion had been performed by Maria Pineda, she insisted that Maria was still doing abortions for other women.

Julian immediately reported this to Dr. Ward Cates and Dr. Carl Tyler. He was first told the CDC had already informed the Texas Department of Health of the facts in the case and could legally do no more, and that, in fact, enough time had been spent on the McAllen case and it should be considered completed. When Julian pressed the matter, stressing that the CDC would look terrible if Maria were to have another death or serious complication, Ward in exasperation told Julian to do whatever he thought was best.

But Julian now had two messages:

Don't do anything; do what you think is best.

Frances insisted Julian immediately call the Texas Department of Health and then report back to us. He agreed and reported: Texas would refer the matter to the appropriate maternal- and child-health committee for investigation.

At least another six months before anything is done, Frances and I decided.

We had to try again. This time we reached higher up in the CDC bureaucracy. Frances called Carl Tyler, the director of the Family Planning Evaluation Division, who in 1969 had put his job on the line for the right to study abortion-related mortality and morbidity. No, not only put his job on the line, but devised a way to carry out the study within the CDC guidelines.

I listened to her exhausting two-hour conversation with Tyler. He was charming, complimentary, concerned but adamant. It was not the job of the CDC to take any action whatsoever in relation to factors in Texas that led to Rosie's death. Yes, they were supposed to identify and eliminate preventable mortality and morbidity due to abortion, but elimination did not imply action. They had informed the Texas Department of Health; it was now up to Texas. Yes, he understood that Texas was not likely to do anything at all and certainly not quickly. He did not know when they would call Texas again to remind them of the case. It would be counterproductive to push too hard. Texas was a difficult state with which to work, and they were not about to jeopardize their relationship.

No, they did not have a protocol to follow when they discovered an illegal act. He did not know why the CDC had not written letters to the various publications *(Ob. Gyn. News, Washington Post, Boston Globe, New York Times)* correcting their stories that Rosie had her abortion in Mexico seeking "privacy." Since February the CDC had known the abortion was directly related to the restriction of federal Medicaid funds.

Yes, Tyler stated, if it were a contagious disease they could quarantine the source. But abortion was not a contagious disease and Maria Pineda was not a carrier. Tyler was now arguing the very opposite of the original rationale that he and his colleagues had used in order to investigate abortion-related mortality and morbidity. It now seemed that unwanted pregnancy was not a sexually transmitted disease.

It became painfully clear that, were any changes to occur in McAllen, Frances and I would have to take action. That evening, when Diane and Pauline came to La Posada, we made our plans. And the next day I took part in the arrest of Maria Pineda.

AFFIDAVIT*

THE STATE OF TEXAS

COUNTY OF HIDALGO

Before me, the undersigned authority a Notary Public in and for Hidalgo County, Texas, on this day personally appeared Frances Kissling, who after being by me duly sworn, upon her oath deposes and says:

My name is Frances Kissling and I am 34 years old having been born on June 15, 1943, in New York City, N.Y. . . . I am managing partner in Reproductive Health Consultants. . . .

I wish to state that on Sunday, June 4, 1978, I arrived at McAllen International Airport, in order to complete research regarding the death of Rosie Jimenez, as a result of an illegal abortion alleged to have been performed by Maria Pineda. With my colleague, Ellen Frankfort, I contacted a number of women in the community who indicated that Maria Pineda was still performing abortions. At this time I would like to state that Ellen and I are presently staying at the La Posada Hotel # 124.

In addition, I called the Center for Disease Control in Atlanta, Georgia, and was informed that a woman in McAllen had reported to them that Maria Pineda was still performing abortions.

On Wednesday evening, June 7, 1978, I went with two Mexican-American women to Maria Pineda's house. Ellen Frankfort and I remained in our car about a half block away while the two women posing as mother and daughter went into Maria Pineda's house and requested an abortion. I only know the first names of the two women; Diane and Pauline. When Diane and Pauline emerged from the house, they informed us that Maria

---

*Errors in transcription in this and the following affidavit have been corrected.

Pineda had agreed to perform the abortion for $125.00 in cash. Diane and Pauline agreed to return to Maria's house at such time as an appointment could conveniently be made. On Thursday, June 8, 1978, we met with a woman named Marta who claimed to know Maria Pineda, and was willing to accompany Diane at the time of the attempted "abortion." Pauline called Maria on Thursday evening, June 8, 1978, and made an appointment for Friday, June 9, 1978, at 1:30 P.M. Accompanied by Chuck Duncan and the cameraman from the ABC affiliate in Dallas, Texas, Ellen, Diane, Marta, Pauline, and I went to the vicinity of Maria's house. Posing as Diane's friend, Marta and Diane entered Maria's house at approximately 1:35 P.M. Diane carried with her $125.00 of my money which I had marked with my initials written on the back side of the bills. Marta had a concealed microphone attached to her bra. Pauline listened to the ensuing conversation between Maria Pineda, Diane, and Marta, which took place in Spanish. At one point, Pauline informed me that Maria told Diane to remove her clothes, that she was ready to perform the abortion. Since Diane had indicated to me that she was willing to go to any length to confirm that Maria Pineda was an illegal abortionist, I felt the situation was now possibly dangerous to Diane's life. I ran to the nearest telephone and called the McAllen Police Department and I identified myself by name. I stated that an illegal abortion was in progress at Maria's house. I gave the street address, stated that the situation was an emergency and that I was afraid the woman, "Diane," would not be able to get away from the house without having an illegal abortion. I stressed that the police should come immediately. I hung up the phone, went outside, noticed the name of the cross street, Hackberry, and called the police back and gave them that cross street. I was then asked to spell my last name, which I did. I waited on the street corner until the police car arrived, which was only about 2–3 minutes. I got into the police car with the police officer and pointed out the house, telling him that he had to hurry [since] as far as I knew the abortion was then in progress.

The above is true and correct to the best of my knowledge and recollection and I give it of my own free will.

Frances Kissling

SWORN TO AND SUBSCRIBED BEFORE ME on this the 9th day of June, A.D. 1978.

NOTARY PUBLIC IN AND FOR
HIDALGO COUNTY, TEXAS

AFFIDAVIT

THE STATE OF TEXAS

COUNTY OF HIDALGO

Before me, the undersigned authority a Notary Public in and for Hidalgo County, Texas, on this day personally appeared Diane* who after being by me duly sworn, upon her oath deposes and says:

My name is Diane and I am 25 years old having been born on August 4, 1952, in Robstown, Texas. . . . I am a student at Pan American University.

I would like to state that the last week of September of 1977, my friend Rosie Jimenez told me she was pregnant and she didn't have enough money to go to a medical doctor for an abortion. We talked about it and we thought that maybe it was just a late period so we went to Reynosa to get a shot so her period could start. Of course it didn't work since it wasn't a late

---

*All last names of local women have been deleted.

period, she was really in fact pregnant. She then decided she was going to have the abortion in Reynosa. I tried to talk her out of it, I wanted her to see her regular doctor. She didn't want to because she said it would cost her $230.00 and she didn't have the money and she was on welfare. I then told her we could raise it somehow, since we were starting school and we were supposed to get some financial help from school. She went ahead and had the abortion, and then I found out she was already in the hospital dying. After Rosie died, at a later date, I found out that Evangelina,** Rosie's friend, had gone with her to Mrs. Pineda's house to have the abortion and that Evangelina had been present when the abortion was done. We found [out] all of this when [Evangelina] told Rosie's future sister-in-law, Pauline, that she had gone with her and had been present at the abortion. When I was advised of this, I called Ellen Frankfort, in New York, since she had already been down to conduct an investigation on Rosie's death. I advised Ellen that I knew the lady who had done the abortion on Rosie. She said she would be down in a couple of days.

Later she and a couple of doctors, one from Austin and one from Atlanta, came down to interview her (Mrs. Pineda) but were unable to get anything out of her. So they went back. During that time she kept calling them to see if anything had been done, and the doctors replied that they were not able to do anything, so Ellen got impatient and came down with Frances on Wednesday, June 7, 1978. Ellen and Frances contacted me and we got together and we decided to [do] something ourselves, since nobody else had.

Wednesday the same date, Pauline and I went to Mrs. Pineda's house and Pauline posed as my mother and told Mrs. Pineda that I needed an abortion and for her to keep quiet. Mrs. Pineda asked who had referred her to us, and we just made up a name. She then said it was $125.00. We told her we didn't have it and that we would come back some other day. She told us to call her for an

---

**Some first names have been changed. See note under Credits.

appointment. We called her for an appointment for today, June 9, 1978, at 1:30 P.M.

On the evening of June 8, 1978, Pauline, Frances, Ellen, Marta and I got together at La Posada and planned everything. We planned that Marta would be wired with listening devices and that the rest of the people (news reporters from Dallas), would be in the station wagon at the corner waiting for a signal to call the police.

On June 9, 1978, Marta and I had the appointment, so we went to Mrs. Pineda's house. She told us to go in and have a seat because she had another patient. We waited until the other people left, then we went into the bedroom; she locked the door and she asked if I was ready. We then started asking her questions on exactly what she would be doing since I was scared and needed to be reassured. She explained what every instrument was for and went into detail on the abortion procedure. She even gave me the name of the shot she was going to give me. I told [her] I was scared and she told me not to worry. She reassured me and said that all she was going to do was put a small red rubber hose in me and that I would start bleeding by tomorrow. She told me not to go to any doctors because they would ask questions, that if I had any complications to go to her and she would give me medicine for pain and infection. She emphasized several times not to go to a doctor should I have complications and that, if I did have, to just say that I had the abortion in Reynosa.

After this she asked me to take my clothes off. At this time the people in the station wagon listening were supposed to call the police. I asked Mrs. Pineda to use her bathroom to stall for time for the arrival of the police. When the police arrived, she was still wearing the gloves. She closed the door on the policemen as they were trying to get into the house. Mrs. Pineda shoved me into the bathroom along with her instruments. At this time I saw her put the little red hose into her bra with a gauze box. Then the officer asked what was going on and I told him we had set her up to perform the abortion. Then he said to get dressed and I got dressed and went outside. I was later transported to McAllen Police Department in an unmarked car.

The above is true and correct to the best of my knowledge and recollection and I give it of my own free will.

<u>Diane</u>

SWORN TO AND SUBSCRIBED BEFORE ME on this the <u>9th</u> day of <u>June</u> A.D. <u>1978.</u>

NOTARY PUBLIC IN AND FOR
HIDALGO COUNTY, TEXAS

As police cars careened around corners, blocking the street to ordinary traffic, and residents poured out to watch the men in blue charge into the lavender bungalow, there was a moment when it seemed we were back on the old frontier.

It didn't last long. As I stood near the door to Maria Pineda's house, now blocked by cops and cameras, Diane emerged and collapsed in my arms. I could feel her entire body shaking. Her back was as drenched with sweat as my own. Whatever distance I had maintained until now dissolved. I was at the house where Rosie had the abortion that killed her, watching the police carry out filthy instruments in kidney-shaped pans.

No longer was I the writer; no longer was Rosie a symbol and Maria a villain. As Diane and I stood embracing, the moment transcended blame. We knew that what had happened to Rosie could, at some point, happen to any of us. We were in the grip of those elements of life we could not always control. And we were one.

AFTERWORD

by Frances Kissling

It has never been my style to call on the police to solve any problem, let alone public health problems. Nor was it a pleasant experience to participate in—no, to actually arrange for—the arrest of Maria Pineda. It may sound exciting; it was sordid. I did not like watching blue-helmeted police converge on Maria Pineda's house, the dogs barking, the news crew angling for the best shots.

It was especially painful to watch and understand the intensity of the experience for Diane, who had agreed to relive her best friend Rosie's final attempt to free herself. Just before she went into the house Diane told me: "You know, if I have to actually have the abortion to stop Maria Pineda, I think I can do it." When Diane came out of the house, she could finally release that control. She had done something for Rosie.

Pauline, who is known in the neighborhood, stayed away from the camera's eye and observed the proceedings from a slight distance.

When Diane, Ellen, Marta, and I were finally released from the McAllen police station, we were drained. For six hours we were questioned individually and threatened with arrest—Ellen, for withholding evidence when she and the Dallas crew would not hand over the videotape; and all of us, for being co-conspirators in an illegal abortion. We felt the need to be together and phoned

Pauline to see if she could join us. She was not in the mood to dine out. "I know it's right that Maria Pineda is no longer practicing," she said, "but I can never feel good to see someone arrested."

Ellen and I understood. We, too, had reservations about the arrest. We have both been strong supporters of the increased use of midwives, not only as an advance in the women's health-care movement, but also because of their traditional cultural importance in the lives of many women. We support the training of more midwives and the retraining of the older midwives.

Yet Maria Pineda did perform the abortion that led to Rosie's death. And that abortion was clearly not an act of mercy. She asked for $125, accepted $100—$25 more than Rosie would have had to pay if she had only known of the San Antonio Reproductive Services Clinic, where a woman on public assistance is charged $75 for a safe, legal abortion. In spite of her years of experience, Maria used primitive and dangerous techniques. Most seriously, in an effort to protect herself, she gave possible fatal follow-up instructions: "If you have any serious problems or complications *don't* go to a doctor or the hospital, come back to me."

Maria Pineda represented a serious threat to the health of women in McAllen. The same false criteria that led to our viewing Rosie as a "poor Chicano woman" could have prevented us from acting to stop Maria Pineda from continuing to do abortions. Maria Pineda needed training, not investigating. Yet there was no way she could receive that training. The health establishment in Texas wants to get rid of the midwives, not upgrade their skills and license them.

The issues were complex, and we needed Pauline and Diane. Their knowledge and feelings about Maria Pineda helped us determine what to do. They guided us in pursuing the arrest as they had helped us learn the truth about Rosie.

As eastern, middle-class, abortion activists, we were limited in what we knew. Initial negative reports from the federal (CDC) investigators in McAllen deterred us from pursuing Rosie's story. Traditional abortion groups—essentially white and middle-class —learned that she might not be a sympathetic figure. She was a

Mexican-American, an unwed mother in a border town noted for illegal drug traffic, and she apparently had been pregnant several times before. In addition, we had been predicting that the restriction of federal funding for an abortion would lead to large-scale mortality and morbidity. But all we could point to was a single death. The decision was made to let Rosie rest in peace, to have a simple memorial service and move on to more significant issues, not human anecdotes.

It took Ellen Frankfort and the women of McAllen nearly four months of investigative work to unearth the full story of Rosie's life and death. When Evangelina stepped forward in February 1978, and identified Maria Pineda as the abortionist, the federal investigators from the CDC were immediately told their first reports were wrong.

They returned to McAllen and conducted taped interviews with Evangelina; they even paid a visit to Maria Pineda, who of course denied her involvement. And with tapes and records neatly deposited in their briefcases for proper storage in the Atlanta CDC files, they returned home to produce a single three-paragraph update on Rosie's death. It appeared on the last page of the March 3, 1978, *MMWR*.

The truth was known and the case was closed to everyone's satisfaction. The CDC, Carter, Califano, the Texas Department of Health, proabortion forces, the local Planned Parenthood, McAllen's doctors and police—all could breathe sighs of relief.

No one seemed to notice that nothing had changed. But that gnawing doubt still in the minds of Rosie's best friends, Pauline and Diane, inspired Ellen and me to continue. They also helped us to realize that ultimate change is not made by institutions or organizations, but by people. We knew that Rosie's death could be used as an excuse for inaction—"Well, she's dead. What more can we do?" Perhaps it is difficult to relate to a dead woman.

And yet, when Marla Pitchford, a Bowling Green, Kentucky, student, tried to abort herself by inserting a knitting needle into her cervix, she was turned over to the police by the doctors she went to for help when the self-induced abortion failed. She was

charged with manslaughter (of the fetus). That charge was
dropped and she was tried on charges of criminal abortion with
a possible sentence of up to ten years in prison. Subsequently,
Marla Pitchford was acquitted on grounds of temporary insanity;
the judge said that even a "quack in a shack" would not face so
harsh a sentence.

The double standard surfaced again in the fall of 1978, when
Marianne Doshi, a college-educated young lay midwife, delivered
a baby girl who died five days after she was born with a knotted
umbilical cord. The midwife acted responsibly and rushed the
baby to a hospital after the complicated delivery. She and the
mother and child were white and middle-class. Hence, the authorities showed none of the supreme indifference exhibited by
Texas, the CDC, and HEW, when a Hispanic midwife became
responsible for the death of a Hispanic mother.

Midwife Doshi was tried for first-degree murder in December
1978. On October 12, 1978, Maria Pineda was sentenced to three
days in jail and ordered to pay a one-hundred-dollar fine.

The baby Doshi delivered could have died even if a medical
doctor had delivered it. It is because Doshi chooses to practice
medicine in an alternative way that she is left vulnerable. And it
is her class and color that are most threatening to doctors whose
practices depend on retaining women of her class.

Maria Pineda's clientele posed no threat to the McAllen medical establishment. Dan Chester, the doctor who attended Rosie,
did not request any police action against Maria Pineda, nor did
he make any arrangements to perform abortions for poor women
for less than his standard $230 fee, payable in full at the time of
the abortion. Neither the D.A. nor the local police investigated
Rosie's death.

The Hidalgo County Health Department, responsible for su-
pervising Maria Pineda, had made no moves to prevent her from
continuing to perform illegal abortions or to deliver babies under
those dangerously unsanitary conditions. The local Planned Parenthood instituted no educational campaign or any other preven-
tive measures.

None of the national organizations active in maintaining abortion rights (National Abortion Rights Action League, Religious Coalition for Abortion Rights) took any action to bring Rosie's story to the public or to help her orphaned daughter.

CDC, the government agency charged specifically with monitoring the effects of the restriction of federal funds for abortion and generally with the "identification and elimination of preventable mortality and morbidity related to abortion," took no discernible action from its February discovery of the cause of Rosie's death until that day of Maria Pineda's arrest in June.

However, I understood the complexity of their dilemma. They work in a highly charged and politicized atmosphere. They are, after all, a division of HEW under Joseph Califano, an HEW secretary opposed to abortion itself as well as to its public funding. The Abortion Surveillance Branch has also been under constant attack as proabortion by the antichoice movement; thus CDC leans over backward to appear neutral.

The branch is short-staffed and has no budget. In fact, the only project related to the Medicaid cutoff that it has received clearance for is the AMSH (Abortion Monitoring in Sentinel Hospitals) study, a survey of abortion complications in twenty-four selected hospitals throughout the United States.

The CDC officials are medical epidemiologists. Monitoring the effects of a political act, the restriction of funding, is a venture into uncharted waters. The serious complications and deaths related to this restriction are not caused by physical disease, nor the natural complications of surgery, but by social and economic pressures. One must draw a clear distinction between legal- and illegal-abortion deaths, between deaths that result from actual medical complications and deaths caused by forcing women without funds to seek unqualified services. Very few women die from legal abortions.

But when the CDC investigates an illegal abortion, it is dealing not only with "bad medicine," but with a downright criminal act. And, in the end, the CDC is a bureaucracy. Most of the Abortion Surveillance Branch members are career staff, not likely to take major risks, to set precedents, but likely to weigh the consequences of any act so carefully as to become virtually paralyzed.

This paralysis extends to their approach to "nonprofessional" people, as shown by the feeble attempt to interview Marta. Although Julian and Mark stopped by her house, only her brother was home, sitting in a bare room watching TV. He was laconic and they felt awkward in asking for information. Their discomfort was partly personal but also related to the CDC restrictions on questioning "subjects." For example, CDC investigators are not permitted to ask single women questions regarding their use of contraceptives. This policy failed in Rosie's case.

I continued to discuss Rosie's importance with abortion groups through the spring and summer. I was told over and over that people are not concerned about the death of one woman. The death of only one woman would not be a strong enough argument to restore public funding. Most shocking, these comments came from activists in the abortion field. We have become so involved in being rational, in countering the antichoice position with facts and figures on relative safety that we, too, have forgotten the importance of people who die while we debate.

The prochoice movement's dedication to "good statistics" has led it to be protective of the CDC. I have felt considerable pressure from my colleagues in the prochoice movement not to criticize them. The paranoia regarding possible damage to the CDC's reputation reached a peak with the cancellation of a panel on McAllen scheduled for the National Abortion Federation annual meeting on September 26, 1978. Ellen Frankfort, Julian Gold, Ward Cates, and I had agreed to discuss the details of Rosie's story and to identify what should be changed in McAllen and other communities to prevent future deaths. It should be noted that neither Ward Cates nor Julian Gold had ever expressed any reluctance to discuss these needed changes. Such an analysis must take place within the abortion movement if we are to be effective in providing women with safe, legal abortions and in conducting a campaign to restore public funding.

As far as the death of Rosie Jimenez is concerned, it is critical that responsibility be placed wherever it belongs. At this writing, plans are underway to bring the case before the courts, civilly if not criminally. A suit for wrongful death will be filed by Rosie's family. They will charge Maria Pineda; Joseph A. Califano, Jr., the HEW administrator who defined the policy that Rosie's pregnancy was not life-endangering; and HEW as the representative of the United States of America, whose government continues to deny its obligation to provide for the health of its citizens.

Most important, the women of America must let the leaders of this country know that we will not tolerate the death of a single woman from a butchered abortion caused by a lack of funding. For each of us the life of one woman is significant.

APPENDIX

AFFIDAVIT*

THE STATE OF TEXAS

COUNTY OF HIDALGO

Before me, the undersigned authority a Notary Public in and for Hidalgo County, Texas, on this day personally appeared Ellen Frankfort, who after being by me duly sworn, upon her oath deposes and says:

My name is Ellen Frankfort and I am 41 years old having been born on October 6, 1936, in New York, New York. I am a self-employed journalist.

I would like to state that I have been part of an investigation of the death of a 27-year-old McAllen woman who died of complications following an illegal abortion on October 3, 1977. I am writing a book about this story for Dial Press and have been working with an investigative team from the Center for Disease Control, Atlanta, Georgia. I have made three trips to McAllen, Texas, and on my second trip, I interviewed Maria Pineda about the death which I had evidence to suspect she was involved with.

---

*Errors in transcription in this and following affidavit have been corrected.

She denied ever doing abortions. On my third trip, in June, I arranged for two Spanish-speaking women from McAllen to visit Maria Pineda to arrange an abortion. Arrangements were made although there was no plan to follow through with the abortion, only to get evidence that Maria Pineda was still willing to perform them. When this was accomplished, a decision was made to contact the media and law-enforcement agencies simultaneously, with the intention of stopping Maria Pineda from practicing medicine in any way.

Today, June 9, 1978, I was in the car outside Maria Pineda's house when two women—one who had been there two nights before, and a friend—entered the house with the plan to document that Maria Pineda was prepared to perform an abortion. In conjunction with a news crew from Dallas, we wired up one of the women so we would be able to record the proceedings and monitor what was going on inside the house in case there was a need for help before the police arrived.

<u>Ellen Frankfort</u>

SWORN TO AND SUBSCRIBED BEFORE ME on this the <u>9th</u> day of <u>June, A.D. 1978.</u>

NOTARY PUBLIC IN AND FOR
HIDALGO COUNTY, TEXAS

AFFIDAVIT

THE STATE OF TEXAS

COUNTY OF HIDALGO

Before me, the undersigned authority a Notary Public in and for Hidalgo County, Texas, on this day personally appeared Marta,* who after being by me duly sworn, upon her oath deposes and says:

My name is Marta and I am 22 years old having been born on September 26, 1955 in McAllen, Texas. . . . I am unemployed at this time.

I wish to state that sometime in September of 1977, I went to a local doctor here in McAllen, Texas, for an abortion, but the fee was too high and I could not afford it. Instead, I decided to go to a doctor in Reynosa, Mexico, and he wanted $35.00 which I also couldn't afford, so I told him I would come back at a later date. However, he wanted to check me to see how far along I was. He inserted some type of instrument into my vagina for the routine check.

Late that same night, while at home, I began cramping but went to sleep anyway. The following morning, I continued cramping severely and [I was] feverish, so I stayed in bed all day until my brother arrived that night. I had no phone, so my brother called an ambulance from the neighbor's house. Subsequently, I was hospitalized with a tetanus infection and lost the baby.

At this time, I would like to stress that when I went to see the doctor in Reynosa, I did not go there for the purpose of an abortion that day.

Then, in October of 1977, a lady identifying herself as Ellen Frankfort, and another writer whose name I don't recall, came by my residence and questioned me about my bout with the tetanus

---

*The last names of some local women have been deleted.

infection. These people informed me that they were from New York and were doing a story on illegal abortions. I told them my story and they left, stating that they wanted me to contact a Dr. Julian Gold from Atlanta, Georgia, who wanted to talk to me concerning my abortion. I did try to reach the doctor, but never got an answer.

On or about the first week in June of 1978, I received a telephone call from Dr. Chester's nurse here in McAllen, and she told me that Dr. Julian Gold had contacted them, and he wanted me to call Dr. Gold collect. I placed the call to Dr. Gold and spoke to him. He said that he was interested in questioning me about my tetanus infection and [whether] Maria Pineda was involved in any way, and I told him that she was not.

Yesterday, June 8, 1978, at approximately 4:30 P.M., a lady who had previously visited with me in October with Ms. Frankfort, came by my house. This lady's name is Pauline. She then informed me that Ellen Frankfort and Frances Kissling were in town and wanted to talk to me. Pauline and I then went over to La Posada, where they were staying. The three questioned me about Maria Pineda and asked if I had any information concerning her illegal abortions. I was then told that they had another girl from Edinburg whose name is Diane and that she was the best friend of Rosie Jimenez, who had died from an illegal abortion performed by Maria Pineda. Diane knew a witness to that abortion, they claimed.

I was then asked if I would like to go to Maria Pineda's residence with Diane to see about an abortion, [for] which an appointment date had already been set for Diane. I agreed to go and they then called a news media in Dallas and informed them about our abortion appointment. I was told that Diane was not pregnant, but that Maria Pineda did not know it and just assumed she was.

Today, June 9, 1978, I was picked up by Frances at my residence, so I could meet the camera crew who had come in from Dallas. The approximate time on this was 9:30 A.M. We went to the hotel room at the La Posada where I was to be wired for the alleged abortion. I also carried a tape recorder in my purse to make sure everything would be recorded.

At approximately 1:28 P.M., we all met at Rivas Food Store, located at Hackberry and 19th, where the camera crew was to be stationed to film our entrance into Maria Pineda's residence, located at 905 North 19th Street. At exactly 1:30 P.M., Diane and I entered her residence. We waited for a few minutes because she was busy, and after a while we were called into a bedroom where she was to perform the abortion. Diane asked her about the procedure and she explained it in detail. Meanwhile, our code to contact the Police Department was that when Maria Pineda asked Diane to take her clothes off, the police would be notified. We kind of stalled for a while, using the excuse that Diane was nervous, so we could give the police enough time to get there and get Maria Pineda performing the alleged abortion. During this time, Maria saw one of the cameramen pass by the window and she asked us what was going on. She quickly removed the rubber gloves from her hands and walked over to the door. By this time, officers were already inside the house. When asked by the officer what was going on, she stated nothing, and [she] attempted to close the door. I opened the door and when the officer asked me what was going on, I told him that I had a recorder attached to my body and that Maria Pineda was attempting to perform an illegal abortion. The officers then placed us in unmarked units and we were transported to the McAllen Police Department.

The above is true and correct to the best of my knowledge and recollection and I give it of my own free will.

Marta

SWORN TO AND SUBSCRIBED BEFORE ME on this the 9th day of June A.D. 1978.

NOTARY PUBLIC IN AND FOR
HIDALGO COUNTY, TEXAS

Epidemiologic Notes and Reports

Cluster of Abortion-Related Complications—Texas

In the period August 8–October 14, 1977, 5 women with septic complications following abortion were admitted to a south Texas hospital. One of the women died with septicemia and renal failure; *Clostridium perfringens* organisms grew from a blood culture.

A review of the hospital records at the 270-bed community facility revealed that only one case of septic complications following abortion had been admitted during the previous year; 2 more women had had such complications but were not admitted (Figure 1). Further investigation indicated that, according to patient or family interviews, all 5 women had had abortions in Mexico. All were of Hispanic descent; 4 were U.S. citizens.

FIGURE 1. *Cases of illegally induced abortion complications, McAllen, Texas, October 1976—October 1977*

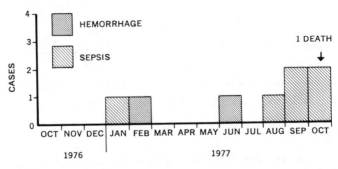

Endometrial and/or blood cultures from 3 of the women grew *C. perfringens* organisms; a fourth patient had tetanus. Three patients were Medicaid recipients. Details of the fatal case follow.

A 27-year-old woman was hospitalized September 26, 1977, with symptoms of fever, knee pain, and lower abdominal pain. She had had 1 previous live birth (in 1973) and 1 abortion (1975). On September 1 and September 19 she had consulted her physician about sternal pain. On the second visit, when she indicated to her physician that she might be pregnant, he informed her that Medicaid no longer paid for abortions. She subsequently obtained an induced abortion in Mexico. On September 26 she was hospitalized. On admission she had a temperature of 101.8 F, with a blood pressure of 110/80 and a pulse of 110. Her uterus was markedly tender and was not easily examined because of abdominal guarding. *C. perfringens* organisms were grown from blood and endometrium. On September 27 a hysterectomy was performed to remove the focus of infection. Her condition continued to deteriorate, however, and she died October 3 from renal and cardiac failure. On October 18, her private physician notified CDC of this death, and, at the request of the Texas Department of Health Resources, an investigation was conducted.

Reported by O Borrundes Falcon, MD, Coordinated General Services of Public Health in the States, Mexico City; R Vargas Machuca, MD, Coordinated Services, Tamaulipas State, Vittoria City; G Perales de la Garza, MD, Health Center, Reynosa, Mexico; B Velimirovich, MD, Pan American Health Organization, El Paso, Texas; FL Duff, MD, C Price, MD, CR Webb Jr, MD, State Epidemiologist, Texas Dept of Health Resources, Abortion Surveillance Br, Family Planning Evaluation Div, Field Services Div, Bur of Epidemiology, CDC.

Editorial Note: This is the first confirmed illegal abortion-related death reported to CDC since February 2, 1976, when a death occurred in El Paso, Texas. Since 1970, however, CDC has investigated 4 other clusters of abortion-related complications. Mexican public health authorities have been informed of the recent cluster and have initiated their own investigation.

Not all states have discontinued public financing of abortions, but Texas law requires that publicly financed health services be partially supported by federal funds. Therefore, by law, Texas withdrew financial support for abortions after federal support was withdrawn on August 4.

While this case was reported to CDC by a private physician, CDC is presently monitoring abortion-related morbidity and mortality through a sentinel hospital system both in states that have stopped funding abortion and in those which are continuing it.

—*MMWR: Morbidity and Mortality Weekly Report* November 4, 1977

Follow-up on Abortion-related Complications—Texas

After the initial report of 5 women who were admitted to a South Texas hospital in a 2-month period with complications following illegally induced abortion *(1),* a surveillance system was initiated to monitor prospectively further abortion-related morbidity in the region. During the 4-month period October 15, 1977—February 14, 1978, 2 additional women were identified with febrile complications after abortion. This figure is consistent with the incidence of febrile complications which occurred before the initial report. One of the 2 women had obtained her abortion in Mexico; both were U.S. citizens of Hispanic descent. Both had uneventful recoveries after antibiotic treatment and uterine curettage to remove retained products of conception.

Further investigation was undertaken of the woman who died on October 3, 1977, from septic complications of abortion. Medical records revealed that she had had at least 2 prior pregnancies terminated by legally induced abortion in the United States. The first abortion was in 1975, the second in 1977. Both abortions were financed by Medicaid funds. She became pregnant again in September 1977. Interviews with the patient's family and a close friend revealed that she subsequently went to Mexico at least once to have an abortion induced by intramuscular injections of unknown agent(s). According to an interview with another close friend, when this method was unsuccessful in terminating the pregnancy, she contacted a lay midwife in the United States to induce the abortion. One day later she had symptoms of fever and lower-abdominal pain. She was hospitalized for *Clostridium perfringens* sepsis on September 26, 1977, and died 8 days later from renal and cardiac failure.

Reported by E Frankfort; D Chester, MD, McAllen, Texas; CR Webb, Jr, MD, State Epidemiologist, Texas Dept of Human Resources; Abortion Surveillance Br, Family Planning Evaluation Div, Field Services Div, Bur of Epidemiology, CDC.

Reference
—MMWR: Morbidity and Mortality Weekly Report March 3, 1978

ACKNOWLEDGMENTS

This book is a collaboration. It could not have been written without help.

Frances Kissling told me of Rosie's death as soon as she found out, and throughout the investigation she kept me informed of the government's activities.

The women of McAllen, invisible to government investigators, told me the real story. This book is dedicated to Pauline, Diane, Margie, Evangelina, and Marta. (For their protection, their surnames are not used; in certain cases—Margie, Evangelina, Rosie's daughter, the nuns, Hortensia, Carmelita, José, and Joey—first names have been changed.)

Juan Chavira, a sociologist at Pan American University, Edinburg, Texas, generously shared his insights into Mexican-American culture in the lower Rio Grande Valley and was the key link to the women of McAllen.

Chuck Duncan of WFAA-TV, Dallas, reported graphically on illegal Mexican abortions and flew down quickly with a crew when asked to cover the arrest of Maria Pineda. He responded to a delicate situation with sensitivity and tact.

Martha Stuart, independent video producer, graciously allowed us to use her videotape equipment.

Mary Mangan encouraged me to point out the inequities of Rosie's death on her WNYC-TV program.

Joyce Johnson, executive editor of Dial Books, exhibited patience throughout the many changes this book underwent. Through her direction, Rosie's story will not live just on videotape and in magazine articles but has been preserved in book form.

Berenice Hoffman gave me the rare kind of encouragement and insights every writer wishes from an agent in helping a general proposal become a specific book.

Certain people, usually anonymous, are essential to a book. Mary Ann Gauger helped type the manuscript, turning scribbled insertions into a smooth typescript; Associate Editor Anita Feldman of Dial has kept track of the book's numerous permutations; and Margaret Wolf did a splendid job of copyediting, adding essential last-minute refinements.

The women at *MS.* magazine, especially Robin Morgan, Suzanne Levine, and Mary Thom, showed a keen interest in making the political implications of Rosie's death known—with a summary and analysis of the events in the January 1979 issue.

Dr. Moshe Hachomovitch, my gynecologist, reminded me, through his competence and compassion during the preparation of this book, that not all doctors are indifferent to women's rights.

Eve Leoff accompanied me on the first two trips to McAllen and shared her perceptions of the Texas landscape through voice and camera.

Sitting down to write a book, even with the help of so many, is solitary work. But I did not write in a vacuum. The Feminist Writers' Guild provided a community of support. And my close friends—Leah Fritz and Marsha McCreadie of the Guild, and Mary Lou Shields and Carol Calhoun—gave me the nurturing every writer needs.

Two people have been special. Hal Davis is one. Just when I was overwhelmed by the complexity of the material and faced a crucial deadline, the New York newspaper strike intervened. Thus Hal could enter the collaboration. With an obsessive love for detail, he helped research the facts, helped rewrite some awkward passages, constantly challenged my conclusions—"Ellen, do you *really* know that?"—and, with a fortuitous combination of journalistic, literary, and editorial talent guided by humane instincts, helped me to place Rosie's death in its proper philosophical frame.

The other was Wesley David Miller, Jr. He was there with the warmth I needed and the understanding that comes with a loving friendship.

—Ellen Frankfort

In addition to the above individuals acknowledged by Ellen, I would like to thank a few others who have been especially supportive of my work on the book:

Myron Chrisman of Reproductive Services, San Antonio, Texas, a founder of the Rosie Jimenez Fund, has quietly been providing poor women in Texas with low-cost or even free abortions and has spoken out against the injustices women still suffer in Texas.

Harriet Pilpel read the manuscript in its later stages and, despite some political reservations, encouraged the telling of this story as it really happened.

Joan Dunlap of the J. D. Rockefeller III Office and Ann Murray of the Hewlitt Foundation have worked to humanize and politicize the abortion issue; both recognized Rosie's story as central.

—Frances Kissling

The Rosie Jimenez Fund

A special fund has been established in the memory of Rosie Jimenez. The fund will provide financial assistance to poor women in Texas who seek abortions. It will also help to make Rosie's story known throughout the country and provide for the education of her daughter.

The fund is tax-exempt. Contributions may be sent to the Rosie Jimenez Fund, 8606 Village Drive, San Antonio, Texas, 78217.

Five percent of the royalties from this book will be contributed to the Rosie Jimenez Fund